SUN DREAMS

SUN DREAMS

SHORT STORIES BY

ROBERT REA

MapleLand Press
Bracebridge, Ontario, Canada

Cover Paintings: Richard Robinson
                  1030 Dickie Lake Road
                  R.R.#1 Baysville, Ontario
                  Canada P0B 1A0

Canadian Cataloguing in Publication Data

Rea, Robert, 1964–
    Sun dreams

ISBN 0-9686997-1-5

    I. Title

PS8585.E3218S96 2001   C813'.6   C00-933252-9
PR9199.3.R42S96 2001

Published by MapleLand Press
Printed in Canada
First Trade Paper Printing: June, 2001

NOTICE:

The author wishes to acknowledge the entire Buwalda family of Beaumaris and surrounds for their help, encouragement, and tolerance through his rather humble and disorganized beginnings.

Narrator's Foreword

"Stories are to a land as facets are to a diamond," Lorna Steinberg was fond of saying. "Each may reflect from a different angle, but all lend sparkle to the same precious stone."

Such words she typically offered on a Sunday when, sitting on her back porch with any willing traveller, this elegant, elderly woman would listen to and discuss stories of homelands near and far. She had engaged in this pastime most of her life, and in both her work as a journalist and in her basic appreciation of life she found the rewards invaluable. Not only did she experience the varied riches of particular regions but gained insights into truths concerning all lands, including her own. Indeed, another favourite saying: "Tell me a story of your home and I will also hear a story of mine."

Sadly, dear Lorna is no longer with us, but out there surely exist others like her, and perhaps you are one. Please consider the book you are now holding. In it are gathered stories from a land called Muskoka — a district in central Ontario, a nook in the great expanse of Canada, a speck in the immensity of the world. The narrator hopes you will enjoy and ponder the presented facets of this land, as Mrs. Steinberg would, in both a specific and general light. Muskoka is perhaps as common as it is unique; it sparkles in ways you may find familiar.

1

The Guests

You could spot BlueberryMuffins a mile away, Doris Stanford always contended. Forever in hiking boots, forever picture-taking, forever sorry when hindering the path of anyone's spit. These were the cherries; at worst they'd dog-ear the main room's wildflower guide. GrandGazers, older and less nimble, were also an easy tag but somewhat more work; the deck chairs were never quite comfortable enough, the lake view never as lovely as in the brochure. Coners were rarely a bother after check-in, the shop windows all in town. Respectively, the business cell phones, speedboat tales, and professional chortles of Getaways, BlurCruisers, and BrownNotes made these among the noisiest; distribution was the key here. As for kids, trade-offs existed. Dirty knees and a bulldozer spelled a Progresser and an extra hour vacuuming, while a good supply of CanoedBefores meant time saved watering dockside flowers. Then again, you might make several trips a season to emerg' with a teenaged WannaSeeMe. But alas, Doris could go on for a month. Why did they come? Her index was both thick and complete. Lord, you could expect that after thirty-three years.

Stanford Lodge, fourteen rooms and twelve cabins united, enjoyed a decidedly privileged location in Muskoka. Set atop a breezy ridge boasting a pleasing mix of beech, hemlock, and yellow birch, it overlooked a tiny and equally pleasing Feather Lake, with plenty of wildlife-rich forest and marsh surrounding all. Jim and Doris Stanford considered this spot ideal for the lodge they'd long dreamed of owning, and in the spring of 1964 they built that dream. Their hunch proved a good one; Stanford became popular, and from spring through fall modestly accommodated souls hailing from Kingston to Korea. "Enjoy and be Enjoyed" read a hand-crafted sign in the lodge's main room, and the message was heeded often.

In response to this success Jim Stanford naturally protected his treasure. He did so, however, in as gentle and humble a manner as he could muster. Though strong in body and mind he was truly a pushover in addressing the demands of guests, and during conversation with the same was invariably bartender-like, never taking a hard stand on any issue. "A noisy camp is a hungry camp" or "A well-fed man never crosses the chef" were typical defences when, during supper, that precious daytime half-hour the Stanfords spent alone, his wife challenged his passiveness. Raised in a poor family he remembered all too well that side of the fence; he would now quietly 'enjoy and be enjoyed' all the way to the bank, thank you.

In contrast, Doris Stanford 'guarded the fort' rather more aggressively. Although frail and unimposing, sixty-something and graying, she compensated with sheer vigilance. To begin, she had the eye of a hawk regarding money, hardly a lodge penny going unaccounted for. Too, residents of nearby communities knew well her fair but strict treatment of employees; senior staff members such as Betty Knowles achieved their status only after many years of hard work and 'unsurpassed service'. But that said, without question Doris's vigilance in protecting the lodge was most apparent in a ritual she indulged in soon after any guest's arrival: 'typing'.

Jim Stanford, when asked by new staff, could never declare exactly when his dear wife began officially branding guests, and for that matter, she herself probably couldn't have either. Her habit was possibly one that seeped into existence rather than sprouted, shifting from her subconscious to conscious musings over the course of decades. No debating, however, its primary function. A novice staff member might suppose it a mere game, a quiet amusement providing relief to long summer workdays. But truly, and as her husband was painfully aware, 'typing' guests was for Doris a devilish approach to maintaining order, and thereby preserving the lodge's fine reputation. Her reasoning was, she argued, quite simple: surmising a guest's primary intention for visiting her lodge, or homeland in general, helped in fulfilling that person's goals. Fulfilling those goals naturally included avoiding conflicts between herself and guests, and between the guests themselves. In strict business terms, of which Doris was fond, her habit allowed her to both 'enhance positives and minimize negatives'. "And call it rude and unfair if you want," she would whisper harshly to her husband, "but it's *working*." To this ultimate result he could scarcely argue; business couldn't have been better, and Doris unquestionably played a major role. At least she never shared her brandings with guests, so despite occasional teasings and remarks of disapproval, as with all else concerning the lodge he would grin and bear.

At the commencement of their thirty-fourth season Jim and Doris remembered little of variation, nor desired it. Their season, with luck, would pass indistinguishable from any preceding it; bookings would be taken, guests would descend in turns upon the lodge, payments would be collected, repairs would be made. They were a mere two years from retirement, and with a buyer already arranged they wanted nothing more than to quietly coast to the finish. And so it was of no small matter when during this otherwise nondescript season, that of 1997, something should occur to upset this peaceful state of affairs.

Elliott and Penny Gibson arrived for a two-week stay on the first Saturday of August that year. The season was at its peak and the Stanfords were more than busy tending to a full lodge. Doris did, however, manage to glimpse this first-time couple outside their car on this morning before they came to reception. The woman, brown-haired and perhaps in her late twenties, had obviously been crying, and her companion, a black-haired, lean fellow slightly older, was apparently arguing with her.

Premature, rude, and otherwise unfair as it may have been, Doris's cerebral Rolodex flipped quickly and harshly. "WorkItOuts," she grumbled to herself. "Here the heck we go."

By the time the couple entered the lodge's rustic foyer Penny Gibson had basically recovered, although her cheeks remained noticeably coloured. Only Elliott Gibson spoke, politely introducing Penny and himself while presenting the confirmation form Doris now cursed herself for faxing out.

"I already assigned you two 'The Wood Duck'," the host proclaimed with a tight smile, lying absolutely. "Our most out-of-the-way cabin. Loads of privacy."

"Sounds perfect," Elliott answered bright-eyed, but all the while glancing at Penny. "Been looking forward to this all winter, haven't we?"

"Yes, this is great," Penny answered almost in a whisper, attempting a smile. At this time Doris noticed darkness under her eyes, and a slight tremble in her hands. The couple's problem, she sadly speculated, was not a new one.

Upon completing the registration she left the Gibsons in the hands of Betty Knowles, then proceeded directly to Jim to report the bad news. She had suffered this sort of problem many times, the experiences painfully etched in her memory. Most notably, there was the young Australian couple six years earlier who half destroyed their cabin during a late-night battle. For two solid hours they had fired every manner of movable object at one another. Similarly the fifty-something couple from Toronto four years earlier who almost burnt their cabin down during a particularly wicked fight; for that incident Doris had even called the police. Countless more could be mentioned. Much as she sympathized with couples having their problems — she and Jim had not been immune — she considered a lodge the wrong place to solve them. It simply wasn't fair to the other guests, she contended, meaning it was plain bad for business.

"They'll get a swift boot home if they cause trouble," Doris declared, arms folded tightly, soon after she found her husband in the workshop. "They're all we needed at this point. A mere season and a half to go and someone just has to rock the boat." She all but spit.

Jim, mending a deck chair broken by one of Doris's LoseAFews, wearily looked up from his work. "Don't doubt you would give them the boot, Doris my love." As often he did when his wife took up her branding iron, he then added a poke of his own. "Sure you've got'em pegged though, Dear? Sure she's not a touch early?"

Doris sneered. "No, I'm *not* a touch early! There's trouble brewing here, and I might remind you it *is* your lodge too, Husband! Maybe it's about time —"

"Yes, I see your point," Jim broke in, blatantly smoothing back thinning gray hair. "I'll go and read the Riot Act to our wonderful guests — sorry, the WorkItOuts — right away." He resumed sanding. "Just as soon as I finish this chair I'll get right on that."

"Super!" Doris replied in a huff, noticing a mischievous grin, and promptly left the room. All on her own as usual, she angrily concluded. The stupid lug would learn the hard way domestic battles had to be avoided.

As things went, however, the Gibsons did not live up to their appointed label. No one working the lodge saw or heard any sign of the couple fighting, and Doris received no complaints concerning them from other guests. "Appears the mighty streak has finally ended," Jim slyly offered at supper one evening, referring to a certain professed record. To this Doris's considerable pride countered with "the jury's still out," but clearly the Gibsons were not living up to her expectations. What pained her even more, however, was a growing suspicion of what truly was the couple's situation.

Doris noticed that anytime she saw the Gibsons together it was Elliott who always led in speaking to others, and who seemed always to decide what the couple did in the way of activities. He was forever giving her orders, if not actually tugging at her arm. For her part Penny seemed totally unenthusiastic about visiting the lodge, or Muskoka in general. She also evidently did not sleep well; every day the couple didn't arrive in the dining room for breakfast until nearly eleven, and always there was darkness under Penny's eyes. What particularly bothered Doris, however, was how the young woman, despite her obvious lack of enthusiasm, seemed very hesitant to utter any protest against her husband. Indeed, the look Doris invariably saw in her eyes did not seem one of anger. It was, rather, of another sort: a look of fear.

Doris's suspicions were only reinforced very early on the Saturday morning of the Gibsons' first week. On Friday night she remained up late cleaning, the kitchen staff member normally responsible for such work being away sick. It was nearly 1 a.m. when she hauled several bags of garbage out to one of the utility sheds. While returning she heard voices from just beyond the start of the lake path, a winding, powdered limestone trail leading downhill some hundred yards to Feather Lake. She managed to identify the sources, partly lit by a nearby driveway lamp. Elliott was holding Penny's arm, and appeared to be drawing her down the path against her will.

Doris quickly ducked behind the shed. She was not close enough to clearly overhear, but occasionally picked up bits of conversation. "You knew it would come down to this," she heard Elliott say, harshly, and later Penny saying, "Please — don't make me do this! Please, Elliott!" Soon, however, Penny stopped arguing, and the two descended the hill.

At breakfast, drawing upon all her strength to stay calm after a nearly sleepless night, Doris politely made inquiries. While the Gibsons took seats in the dining room, arriving late as usual, she approached their table and painfully attempted her best lodge-host smile. "Sleep well?"

A tiny but definite crease formed in Penny's pale brow. With fluttering eyes she looked to Elliott, who answered, "Not so well, quite honestly." He stared at the table a moment before looking up at Doris. "But please don't take offence. Penny and I simply need time adjusting to new places."

"Your cabin's okay?"

"The cabin's great, thanks."

"There's nothing you need? There's ... nothing bothering you?"

Elliott looked out to the driveway, which was busy with the Saturday turnover. "No, we're doing fine. Just fine, thank you."

"The shops in town are lovely," Penny suddenly added, softly. "We're having a good time, Mrs. Stanford." As when first meeting her, Doris noticed a tremble in her hands.

Doris silently stared into her dark eyes a few seconds, awkwardly, then smiled and quietly said, "Well that's great to hear. I'm glad you're enjoying yourself."

Turning back to Elliott she fought to maintain her smile. "Just let me know if there's anything I can do to make your stay more pleasant." With that she trudged back to the main desk. On her way, however, she again glanced at the Gibsons: Elliott was now whispering something to Penny, a fiery look in his eyes.

"I'd like to crack his head open with a frying pan, is what I'd like to do about it!"

This was delivered to Jim soon after he and his wife retired to bed that evening.

"He's definitely mistreating her, and mistreating her badly. I'm convinced now. She may not have bruises or scars — at least none I've seen yet — but she has all the signs of emotional abuse. I've had friends go down that road; I've seen this before."

Jim, closing *Of Golden Years & Golden Hobbies*, which he had long given up trying to read, said, "Yes, I know you have. But keep in mind these aren't friends, Dear. They're customers. And it may sound cold, but we simply can't get involved."

This Doris could not refute. One of the worst mistakes a lodge host could make was to stick his or her nose into a guest's private affairs, especially serious affairs. It was a death sentence for a lodge's reputation, even more damaging than becoming known for hostile or rowdy occupants. And she as much as Jim didn't want their lodging career ending under such a cloud.

"Besides," Jim continued, "You're positive you're not getting the wrong impression with these two? I talked to the fellow for a few minutes one day. Seemed nice enough. He said he was here because he grew up in Muskoka and missed it. He's one of your MemoryLaners, Dear."

"Yeah? Well goody for him! Probably doesn't give a hoot what *she* wants to do. She clearly doesn't want to be here." Doris sighed. "The poor thing — she seems so scared and depressed. She's obviously got herself into a terrible situation."

"Perhaps she has. But promise me, nonetheless, you'll stay out of it."

Jim stared at Doris, and at last she said, "We'll see."

"We'll see?"

Doris again sighed, and begrudgingly offered, "I will."

But she didn't.

The undeniable truth was, at heart she was already involved, and too much so to back away. Every time she laid eyes on Penny Gibson during the days following her feelings of pity toward this young woman, and anger toward her husband, only grew deeper.

Her first opportunity to talk with Penny alone came the following Monday. Seeing Elliott drive away shortly after noon Doris made a trip to their cabin, already armed with the excuse she needed to check some troublesome plumbing.

Penny greeted her at the door with a nervous smile and let her in. Doris immediately noticed she looked very drawn. Nonetheless the young woman proceeded with typical chitchat about the weather and events in town, such as a craft show taking place. For Doris ten gruelling minutes passed before she managed to turn conversation in her desired direction.

As she knelt and inspected the entirely leakless bathroom sink pipes, she said to Penny, who stood at the door watching, "So are you and Elliott honeymooning, if you don't mind me asking?"

Remaining silent a few seconds, Penny answered, "Oh, no. We've been married several years now."

"Ah, but a few years *is* still honeymooning, if you ask me."
Doris turned and smiled at Penny. "Of course, 'honeymooning'
maybe isn't the best word, is it? All considering."

"Considering what?"

Continuing her inspecting, Doris said, "That ... the first few
years are the toughest. I've seen enough new couples in my time,
you must remember."

When Penny didn't respond Doris continued with, "Yes,
believe me, I know. I may have been lucky with Jim, but a few
women in town were definitely not." Doris now turned to Penny.
"Some ran into serious problems, and needed help. I, you see, was
one of the helpers."

Doris uttered her final words with distinct emphasis, and saw
they were duly noted. Penny's eyes noticeably bulged, and she
began fidgeting with the bathroom door handle. With a slight
quiver in her voice she at last said, "Well, thankfully that's not me.
Elliott loves me very much, Mrs. Stanford."

"Doris. Just call me Doris. And that's great —"

"In fact, Elliott bought me flowers yesterday when he was in
town."

Doris turned back to the sink and bit her lip. She wanted to say,
"Sure — probably right before spending double that on a whip."
Oh, she had seen denial many times too; she now felt worse for
Penny than ever.

With the bathroom 'problem' exploited for all it was worth,
and with her guest seemingly uncomfortable, Doris made her way
to the door. While stepping out, however, Penny surprised her.

"You needn't worry at all about me, Doris. I'm fine. I really am."

The two women locked eyes a moment, the elder agonizingly
caught between wanting to jump in head first at this point, and
exercising business caution. Watching Penny, Doris sensed the
young woman was about to say more, and very much wanted to say
more. Too, if she did, Doris could easier justify her involvement;
the guest would be taking the initiative. Ultimately, however, Penny
remained silent.

Exasperated, Doris could only awkwardly reply in a professional tone, "I'm so sorry if I've become nosy. Please accept my apologies." She then quickly turned and headed back to the main lodge.

The next four days only brought Doris more evidence of Penny's suffering. On several occasions more she observed Elliott speaking harshly to his wife, only for her, as usual, to silently acquiesce. The late morning risings also continued, the darkness under Penny's eyes only deepening. For Doris the situation developed to where she herself had difficulty sleeping at night. Often after an hour of lying awake she would slip out the lakeside door and sit awhile on their apartment's tiny second-floor balcony, musing and worrying. And ironically, only because of such a habit did she soon witness something that would make her heart almost stop.

The Friday evening began typically, with Doris retiring to bed at midnight only to rise an hour later and pad out to the balcony. The night was warm and she didn't bother with a sweater. Seating herself she gazed out to the lake and surrounding forest, which were softly lit by a full moon. The lodge and grounds were completely silent save for the occasional faint rustling in the nearby woods.

It was after about a half-hour that Doris heard the sound of light footsteps on gravel, and turned to see Penny Gibson. She was standing at the foot of the path leading down to the lake. She was alone, or at least Doris could not see her husband, and seemed indecisive, almost frantic. Several times she started down the path only to return. Also, each time she entered the swath of the driveway lamp Doris saw the young woman bring her hands to her face, and blatantly wipe away tears. Finally, however, she started down the path, and kept going.

Doris didn't need long to digest what she had seen and suspect Penny's intentions that August night, the Gibsons' last at the lodge. And reputation be damned; this host would not sit back and simply learn in the morning whether her suspicions were correct.

Having gone out to the balcony half-dressed she needed only a few clothes from the bedroom, and with these on, and Jim unstirred, she softly padded out the apartment door. After negotiating a quiet path down the creaky main stairs she stepped out the foyer's side door.

By the full moon's light she managed to follow the lake path without a flashlight. She stumbled several times nonetheless, and each occasion, fearing Elliott might be out looking for Penny and would hear any stumblings, she stopped to listen for him. Although the night was warm, during such pauses she shivered. She also felt her heart beating.

Upon approaching the dock Doris slowed her pace, keeping as quiet as possible. She felt this Penny's most likely destination and wanted to watch her a moment before giving herself away. She might, after all, be entirely wrong about what her guest had in mind.

Stopping at a large pathside pine, she peered out from behind it to the dock, which was lit by a posted lantern identical to that at the head of the lake path. Penny was not in sight, and no sounds came from the lake or surrounding woods. After about a minute she ventured onto the dock and soon confirmed her worry: the young woman was not there.

Only one other possibility lay open, and Doris glanced toward the start of the path that circled the lake. With overhanging tree branches it was much darker than the path descending from the lodge, and she found herself once again shivering. Determined to get to the bottom of this matter, however, and greatly concerned for Penny's welfare, she continued.

The path circling Feather Lake, one the Stanfords made themselves, was stylishly named 'Feather Rendezvous'. Following close to shore, it first took the hiker through stands of pine and spruce and a marshy area at the lake's north end. Ultimately it led to a long, narrow bay on the lake's northwest side. It was this bay giving the lake its name, and the 'rendezvous' to which the path's name referred. Not only did the narrow inlet gradually taper to a point, but from both sides striated bedrock sloped gently down to the centre, and the eventual V delineated the stem of the 'feather'. The bay had become one of the lodge's conversation pieces over the years, and also, being shallow, was a favourite swimming spot for lodge guests with young kids.

When Doris arrived at the bay she was not long in making a discovery, and what she saw took her breath away.

Standing motionless in the shiny, moon-lit water up to her waist was Penny Gibson. She was peering down, and, seemingly, pondering.

Doris was beside herself. She considered calling to Penny, but then thought better of it. She knew from years of experience how well sound carried over the lake, and the last thing she wanted was other guests becoming disturbed or involved, including Penny's devil of a husband. And perhaps being so distracted was responsible for Doris not seeing the devil until he was standing right beside her.

Cupping his hand over her mouth, he whispered in her ear, "Shh. She's almost there."

Not since the summer of '82, when the clothes of a seven-year-old KampKeeper momentarily caught fire, had Doris fainted. This time it was much the same, with her vision slowly fading as she slumped to the ground. Too, when she regained consciousness, and saw Elliott Gibson peering closely down at her, she almost had experience number three.

He was seated on the bedrock, however, gently holding her head in his lap, and his immediate words were soft and soothing. "I'm so sorry, Mrs. Stanford! I didn't mean to scare you, but if I had warned you Penny would have heard, and that might have spoiled everything. She's doing so well tonight — just look at her."

Doris sat up and peered out to the lake, to the spot where she had seen Penny. The young woman was no longer there. Doris soon spotted her, however, the moon offering just enough light. She was swimming, slowly, at the mouth of Feather Bay.

Doris needed time finding her voice, but at last said, "What in the world —?"

"Penny's learning to swim again."

"Swim *again*?"

"And we were hoping not to bother anyone with this."

"What's this?"

"This," came a smartly-delivered answer, "is my little project."

In the quarter-hour that followed Elliott Gibson offered an explanation. All the while he kept an eye on Penny, who swam intermittently. For Doris's part, she paid attention to both these guests, ultimately as puzzled by one as the other.

"Penny's father owned a garage," Elliott quietly began. "Part of the business was looking after trucks broken down on the highway. He had a real fondness for draft horses, and he actually named his big wrecker 'The Silver Clydesdale'. Soon after he bought the truck Penny's mother, Nora, also got licensed to drive it. She thought it'd be handy at times if both she and her husband could drive the wrecker and she proved right. Problem was, she needed to drive it so rarely that when she did she was always rusty.

"One August night Nora drove Penny and me — we'd been dating about two years at that point — home from the garage in the big wrecker because Penny's father wanted to work on the family's pickup. Nora was a strong woman and very capable, but she wound up losing control of the truck that night on a narrow bridge. A car was coming from the other direction and I think she was scared she wasn't giving it enough room. She veered pretty hard to the right just before the car reached us, and that's all it took: we broke through the old railing of the bridge.

"The night was warm so we had both windows open. The cab filled with water quickly. Crazy as it might sound, my first feeling wasn't fear for our lives but worry over the serious trouble we were in with Penny's father. Nora, though, thought only of getting us kids out of the truck. She started screaming at us to climb out the window. This we could only do, though, when the cab was almost completely filled with water. Penny went first and I was right behind her. Nora gave me no choice; she was every bit as strong as me at that age, and she basically kicked at me until I was out the cab window.

"The moon was full that night and it gave enough light for me to see up to the surface. The river was about twenty feet deep where we were, and although that may not sound like much, it seemed an awfully long way up.

"When I finally reached the surface I needed nearly a minute to get my breath back. Penny, luckily, seemed fine. But Nora was nowhere to be seen. I dove down again a few times but it was no use — the river was just too dark and deep. And by the time help arrived, of course ..."

Elliott rubbed his eyes. "Aside from losing her mother, Penny was never the same with deep water after that night. In the first years following the accident, if you took her anywhere near a lake or river she'd start screaming, and you couldn't hold on to her. It was awful. And what was worse, before the accident she had always loved swimming. It was one of her passions.

"Anyway, a few years ago some buddies of mine invited me on a canoe trip down the Black River. During that trip I came up with the idea of bringing Penny to this area. I figured maybe one way to help restore a joy in her life was to push her to meet her problem head on. Maybe with some that approach might be cruel, but I knew from other experiences this was the best with Penny. She might not seem it on the outside, but she's pretty tough.

"Muskoka struck me as the perfect place to give things a try. I grew up here, and I knew you could hardly walk a mile in any direction without encountering water. Penny would have no escape. I thought I'd even try getting her swimming during a full moon, the way it was during the accident. That's why I booked the lodge for when I did. Silly as it might sound, but I wanted to basically 'recreate the crime scene'. As you can see, though, it's worked. It took a serious effort — lots of nights coming down here to the lake, and missing sleep — but Penny's back doing what she always loved."

With his explanation complete Doris remained silent a moment digesting, and regretting. Elliott seemed to read her mind, because he next said, "You didn't think very highly of me, did you?"

Doris tried her best at innocence. "I'm not sure —"

"Don't deny it. You thought I was abusing Penny. She told me about the little talk you two had at the cabin. If you're wondering why she didn't just tell you then about her problem it's because she finds it embarrassing. She's really sensitive about it."

Doris put her hands on her hair. "All I can say is I'm so sorry. It just seemed that ..."

"I know how it seemed, and I'd probably have thought the same. It took some tough prodding to even get Penny to Muskoka, let alone in the water, and I'm sure all of that didn't look very good from a distance." Elliott turned to Doris, and his voice became very soft. "But make no mistake now — I would never do anything to hurt Penny. She's the love of my life, Doris."

Out of the water, that love approached. Not startled by the sight of Doris, she apparently already noticed the lodge's owner. "I see you've found a friend," she said to Elliott.

What followed was yet more explanation by Penny, and the women exchanging apologies. All soon seemed resolved, but then Elliott surprised Doris again on this evening. He did this as Penny waded back into the lake.

"The best part, Honey," he said, "is that Doris says she wants to join us for a late-night dip. Isn't that great?" Before Doris could answer, he once again whispered in her ear. "It would help so much with her confidence. Would you, please?"

This request on its own would not have been enough to push Doris over the top. But then came more incentive. After Elliott delivered his plea his wife looked back toward shore, and for the first time since arriving at the lodge Doris saw, in the soft light of the full moon, Penny Gibson offer a genuine smile.

And so it was that nearing 3 a.m. on a fine August morning in 1997, Doris Stanford, in only the clothes she was born wearing, joined Penny and Elliott Gibson for a swim in Feather Lake.

The event proved almost magical, Doris would later reflect. For a good half-hour, keeping close to shore, the three swam and splashed and behaved generally like kids. Eventually, however, Doris ran out of steam and merely floated on her back, gazing up at the moon and faint stars. At this time she also watched Penny, who by now seemed utterly at ease with the water. Earlier, when her energy was still high, Doris playfully dove underwater some six feet, and while returning to the surface, wanting for air, was chilled by the ghostly, greenish view of the moon. For a few seconds she identified with the horror this young couple went through that fateful night summers ago, and in turn felt very glad for them,

especially Penny. In contrast to earlier she now seemed so happy.
Indeed, Doris's most treasured memory of the young woman on
this night was of her also floating on her back, giggling like a
teenaged girl again, clearly relishing something rediscovered: the
smooth, comforting wonder that is also water.

Doris slipped into bed as quietly as she had slipped out. Slowly
drawing the light blanket to her chin, she closed her eyes. Outside,
birds were chirping. She couldn't bear glancing at the clock.

"So?"

Doris shook at the sound, but soon recovered. Turning to the
source she wearily said, "So what?"

"So what's a head of lettuce go for in Ufford these days?"

Doris ran her hands over her face. "It was nothing, after all."

"Really?" Jim mumbled into his pillow. "That's not what I heard."

Doris's head snapped around. "Not what you —?!"

Jim grinned against her glare. "You weren't as quiet leaving
here as you thought, my dear, and I followed you. To the start of the
path heading to the lake, at least. That's where I ran into the Gibson
fellow."

"You fol— *And*?"

"And he gave me a quick explanation. From there I thought I'd
just leave you to it. Thought maybe ... it would be good for you."

"*Good* for me?! How the heck would it be good for me?"

Jim snickered. "The ol' file ain't quite complete yet, Doris my
love. Even after thirty-three years they're still comin' for things
you've never seen before. Admit it."

"I'll admit nothing."

"What, by the way, are we going to call this new type?
AquaSpooks? MoonLoons? Lak—"

Doris's pillow struck its mark. "They came to simply ... *swim*.
Plain old SplashHounds. And you can shut up now, please."

"Yes, Dear," came a muffled answer, and Doris looked to the
window immediately next to her, where the sun was just rising
behind the lake.

2

A Precious Bend in the River

If paddling this part of Muskoka's north branch on a summer evening you would hear the piano and chorus long before reaching the bend. The music was soft and gentle but carried well along the river. When at last you arrived you would not see the singers, however, nor surmise their number. You would only notice the voices came from within a modest, white house overlooking the bend, and, on perhaps one such evening, these words they brought forth:

> *Let us rise once again,*
> *In the gracious sun of a novel day.*
> *To fairness and peace,*
> *To love and good will,*
> *For each, for all, and forever.*
> *Let us rise once again.*

On an autumn evening in 1995 the river voices were especially strong; the residents of the white house were having a party. As usual with festive occasions trimmings were modest and few, but a shiny maple armchair made an appearance, and so too a candled cake.

"Happy tenth, Sally," a shy young man quietly said to the evening's somewhat dazed star, approaching the piano bench. "I just ... don't know how to thank you." Several tears slowly descended from his eyes.

"Now, now — whether you realize it or not, you thank me every day, Paul," Sally Stanton softly and truthfully replied, gently stroking his hair. Turning, in a louder voice she said, "Happy anniversary to everyone, whatever your years at The Corner!"

This elicited cheers from the others, who numbered seven, and soon they busied themselves carrying food from the kitchen to the decorated dining room table. Sally remained seated at the piano, however, merely watching the group. And when at last she rose she did not immediately join them but went to the house's large front window, to the view of the river below. From that river one could have seen her smile fade. "Ten years — my God," she whispered, her face almost pressed against the glass to conceal it from the others. As with Paul tears ran down her cheeks, but these she quickly wiped. She would be strong on this special night. The others expected and needed her strong and she would not disappoint them. Not at this stage. Ten years had passed now.

If Sally Stanton might somehow have lived her life over she doubted she could have made it unfold differently. Born into a wealthy and very conservative family her destiny, it seemed, was set from the beginning. Sometimes, lying awake at night, she let herself dream of such a second chance, pondering how she might have hidden her 'unacceptable ways', or perhaps even changed herself altogether. But always she was left accepting who she truly was, and how any number of attempts at disguise would not have changed that underlying self, nor any self-manipulation. She was, after all, as visible to herself as to others. She also, most significantly, saw no shame in who she was.

Her first crush came early, when she was only in second grade, and was on a tiny, brown-haired girl named Mandy. Her family had recently moved to Oakville, and Sally often found herself staring at this new girl during class and at recess. She thought Mandy exciting; she was full of surprises, and her eyes, too, were such a beautiful soft blue. Later, when the two girls became friends, they would often visit one another's house after school to play games, or when at Sally's, to try playing her family's grand piano. They also often slept over, and during summer vacations one would invariably join the other's family for trips. The two girls became inseparable. It was, Sally would later fondly reflect, a time of purity and innocence, and one instilling in her forever a belief in the true foundation of all future bondings. Specifically, her attraction to her own gender was innate, and displayed itself long before she had any clue what went on behind bedroom doors.

In the high school years following she had, like everyone during that period, numerous relationships. Similar also, she never intended all such relationships as ever-lasting. This was now a time of abandon, of experimentation. With this came not only a growing awareness of who she was but a growing acceptance. "What was so wrong with 'walking on the other side of the road'?" she began wondering, sometimes out loud. And feeling this way — becoming increasingly liberal and in turn less cautious — undoubtedly was responsible for what happened next. It was inevitable.

In the fall of 1967, one year after she began college, her mother learned. How, specifically, Sally never discovered, but when she arrived home one weekend in November her mother confronted her, red-faced and trembling with anger.

It was a disgrace, Gloria Stanton declared; a monstrous embarrassment to the family. "How can we possibly show our faces in public now?" To this Sally, head lowered, only listened silently. What *could* she say? To begin, she didn't believe her mother could ever possibly understand the filter through which she viewed the world. Second, in denying the rumours she would only confess to perceiving her behaviour as a crime, and she saw no crime. Lastly, if she indeed was a criminal she was hopelessly so; was she to offer, "Sorry, I won't do it again"? She ultimately left for her bedroom that afternoon without saying a single word. She also buried her face in her pillow so her mother wouldn't even hear her crying.

Life for Sally was most definitely not the same after that day. Her parents made it clear they wanted nothing to do with a "disgusting" daughter, and she could either "clean up her act" or be effectively disowned. Most of her fellow students, who curiously also soon found out, became awkward with her if not downright rude. She felt stares from almost everyone when in public. Snickers behind her back also were common, and if she had a stone for every 'dyke' she heard she could have built one. This continued several years. Finally, after her mother refused to answer the door when she tried visiting one cool day in November of 1972, Sally returned to her school dorm, packed up, and left.

So began thirteen years of drifting. Reflecting back on this time Sally sometimes needed a minute to name all the places she lived, all the jobs she had. There was, among many others, the eight-month stint at the car seat factory, the three months as a secretary, the two years at a garden centre, the week and a half dry walling. There was Sarnia, Belleville, Renfrew, St. Thomas, North Bay. Something she didn't have difficulty remembering, however, was her reasons for moving. They were always of the same mix. She felt, or by fellow employees was outright deemed, an outcast, her landlord declared her lifestyle 'inappropriate', or she made the mistake of falling for someone who did not share her sexual orientation. Whatever the particulars, Sally never allowed herself to get overly settled in or attached to a new place when she moved. It might be a few years but then it might be that afternoon she once again pulled up stakes.

During this period, in a fight against depression, she turned to a nearly lifelong interest: music. She was about four when she started toying with her family's piano, twelve when she began playing and singing her own songs. In developing her talent she turned down countless offers from her parents for lessons. Rough or unconventional as her style may have been, it was hers, and she wanted it to remain that way, untainted by the piano teachers she thought all sounded the same. Besides, she knew quite early hers was not to be a particularly conventional life anyway.

Somehow — miraculously, sometimes — she always found a piano she could play. In a restaurant she waitressed the evening shift, for instance, that piano was one stored in a back room, the instrument retired from days when the establishment offered live entertainment. After a rough day, which was almost every day, she would offer to close up, then remain at the piano until the earliest hours of the morning, playing and quietly singing. Her songs were both of mourning and renewal, and any who heard her play — always by accident, for Sally considered her music private — were invariably moved. Her lyrics were simple and even typical, phrases bright and promising, yet set to music hinting of deep despair. A listener was at once inspired and saddened.

It was in April of 1983 that Sally moved to Bracebridge. Up until this time she had been living in Kingston, working as a shipper-receiver in a textile factory. Feeling it was yet again time to move on she acted quickly when hearing from a sympathetic fellow employee about a landscaping job in Muskoka. This fellow's uncle had his own business and was willing to take on inexperienced help. A few phone calls later the job was hers.

She moved within a month, making several trips to Muskoka beforehand to search for an apartment. The one she ultimately took proved no prize, so in the months following, with the landscaping job working out well, she kept her eye on the paper.

As things went, however, it was a lunchtime stroll that led Sally to her next place of residence. Her employer landed a contract to improve the lawns and gardens at a retirement home situated on the north branch of the Muskoka River. Over the weeks at this job she came to love the peacefulness and beauty of the river setting and took to strolling the shore at lunch. It was on such a stroll, and upon reaching a sharp bend a quarter mile upriver from the retirement home, that she came across a real estate sign on an empty lot. Later inquiring with the agent she learned the lot was three acres, and quite a bargain. It drove her to thinking.

She took a closer look at the property the following evening after work. No mystery why it was a bargain. The bending river eddied in front of the lot, and the water here was shallow; in many places bedrock protruded above the surface. The lot itself rose steeply from the river and was boulder-strewn. Sally was nonetheless taken by the setting, finding it even more peaceful than in front of the retirement home. Indeed, no other cottages or houses were in view from this point. What the property lacked could also be considered a blessing — its 'faults' made affordable to her a piece of land that otherwise would not have been. So, deciding to gamble she placed an offer the very next day. What soon followed was about half of Sally's life savings going toward a down payment.

A house was several years in coming. This she at last afforded by having a contractor do only the framing, slowly completing the rest herself. Too, by this time she had taken the plunge and started her own one-person landscaping business, and often there were remnants from the small jobs she took on. Also contributing was the river; the first spring after moving into the house its owner hooked enough passing planks and logs to build herself a crude but sufficient dock.

With such savings, in July of that same year Sally even managed to acquire what she considered the house's final touch: a piano. Old and battered as the school upright may have been, it would more than do. No longer did she need to sneak sessions but could play to her heart's content. Over the remainder of the summer she played more often than the previous fifteen years combined, writing over a dozen songs.

That autumn, her optimism toward the future growing, she allowed herself a private housewarming, fit for one. As part of the festivities she mounted a crude, homemade plaque in the lot's wooded back corner. It sat low to the ground, out of sight from the river, and only someone on foot searching was likely to notice it.

Stanton Corner
May I here rest
May I here 'retire'
October 6, 1985

For several minutes Sally stared at the plaque, then turned and cast her eyes over the lot, the house, and the gently-flowing river. For the first time since leaving her parents she allowed herself she had found what she was looking for, and so dearly needed. A tranquil place, a place belonging to her, and, just maybe, a home at last.

Richard Hastings knew, without the slightest doubt, when the time came he would do it. No one would be at the viewpoint at three in the morning on a weekday, and so no one would be there to stop him. No one could try talking him out of what he desperately needed to do. It would be simple, really. Close your eyes, take one step forward, endure several seconds of cool, rushing air, then all would be over. And little Stacey — clutched in his arms, sound asleep — wouldn't feel a thing. He'd calculated they'd strike the rocky bottom of the cliff at nearly sixty miles per hour, and no one, surely, could survive a fall like that. They would both be killed instantly, and so would end the headaches, the nightmares, the screaming. It was the right thing to do, the only thing to do.

As a teenager Richard would never have fathomed such an end to his life. Full of vigour and grand ideas he saw only pleasant and fruitful years ahead. He would not concede to family tradition and become a mechanic, the occupation of his father and grandfather, but would follow his own star. That star, he felt strongly, would lead him to a civil engineering degree and, eventually, his own firm. Few doubted his ability to achieve such goals; in high school he was gifted in math and physics, and through summer jobs had already demonstrated a talent for business. "He's headed places, this kid," an employer once told Glen Hastings, and although he, like most fathers, initially resented his son shunning his footsteps, he soon became accepting and supportive. Who was he, after all, to hold back a prodigy? For Richard the future could not have looked brighter.

In pursuing his dreams he knew, even at fifteen, he would leave Sydney, Nova Scotia. As much as he loved his hometown and province he was convinced better education and career opportunities in engineering lay elsewhere. When he finished high school he would head west. His only question was: would he venture into the world alone, or with a companion?

It was in 1976, then seventeen, that Richard met Leanne Rowland. He was forcibly paired with this shy but sharp-witted girl for a Ferris wheel ride at an autumn fair. Richard was already somewhat familiar with her; she waitressed part-time at a restaurant he and his father frequented when visiting Cape Breton Island. While chatting on the Ferris wheel he came to know her better, however, and, mutually intrigued, within days of that fair the two began dating.

Richard's fondest memories with Leanne during those early years came from a viewpoint on the Cabot Trail. From this spot they could take in the full sweep of the sea, a sea which for Richard had always symbolized a "path to somewhere else." Everything he ever dreamed of, seemingly, lay across that huge sea. And what he learned during visits to the viewpoint, and what ultimately made them so memorable, was that Leanne Rowland felt the very same way.

Soon after high school the couple married, and within a year moved to Vancouver. Both entered university, Richard in his civil engineering and Leanne in nursing, and both later graduated. Good jobs followed and the couple soon bought their first house, a tidy, two-bedroom in a modest but pleasant neighbourhood. When a tiny Stacey Hastings arrived into the world one November evening a year later Richard and Leanne were beside themselves with delight. They loved the baby wholeheartedly, spent many a day entirely engrossed in her goings-on, and by the time Stacey was five her goings-on were considerable. Together with their careers progressing as hoped the couple wondered that their lives could get much better.

The Hastings' neighbours seemed equally content with their lives. The Jacobs were a family of five, two parents and three teenaged sons. The boys, like Leanne and Richard, were well-educated and seemed destined to live up to their parents' high hopes. Sure they drank and carried on now and then, but who didn't at that age? Richard, especially, enjoyed talking with the boys.

Several blocks from the Hastings' house was a small, tree-lined park the family much enjoyed. They would have picnics, frolic in the playground, watch evening soccer and baseball games. It was a sunny place, an inner-city haven the family treasured and greatly looked forward to visiting. It was also a place where, on a November afternoon of 1986, Leanne Rowland would be raped and murdered.

She and Stacey had been at the park only fifteen minutes when their three teenaged next-door neighbours arrived in a pickup. They parked fifty yards from the playground, where Leanne watched Stacey, and began drinking heavily. Unbeknownst to Leanne, they also began increasingly eyeing her.

When they finally approached she was in the midst of getting drinks from the car. Immediately sensing trouble she shouted to Stacey to stay at the swings. What followed, however, Stacey Hastings witnessed clearly: the boys took turns with her mother, and as she lay half-naked and sobbing on the cold gravel beside the car, her three 'rising star' neighbours slit her throat from ear to ear.

Later — anytime later — Richard Hastings could clearly remember only the two police officers who came to his office that afternoon. Indeed, after several months all he knew was his wife's attackers were never arrested, his daughter remained deeply troubled, and life as the family had known it could never be again.

From the day he received the news Richard became afflicted with a pounding, almost numbing headache that seemed never to go away or even subside. While watching Leanne's casket being carried at her funeral he vomited and collapsed, so intense was his migraine. During the following two months off work he could barely function.

Even worse, however, was Stacey's condition. Every evening she had nightmares, and woke screaming and shaking terribly. Richard tried everything to help her but to no avail. The doctors, too — and he lost count how many he consulted — could offer little. "I'm afraid no one can say when, or if, she'll recover," one quietly informed him. His dear, precious daughter was now living a life of horror.

It was not long before things fell apart with Richard's work, which for lack of savings he was soon forced to resume. While clearly sympathetic, his firm could not extend his grace period indefinitely, and as his late days, missed days, and costly mistakes mounted his termination was inevitable. "Why don't you go back east," his boss tenderly suggested. "Maybe, surrounded by family, you could somehow start again ..."

His boss was not necessarily wrong, Richard knew, but there would be no starting over. All his dreams seemed both crushed and crushed forever. No one could replace Leanne; no one could make him forget Leanne. He was finished.

It was in such despair one night, while holding Stacey almost an hour as she cried and shook in his arms, that Richard turned a corner and formulated a plan. He would take his dear, terribly suffering daughter, and likewise himself, to that same highland viewpoint he and Leanne had so enjoyed together and make it their last view of the world. He would indeed use the "path to somewhere else." Only a railing stood between the sheer cliff and the bench he and Leanne had shared seemingly an eternity ago; it would not be difficult. He'd make a trip out east, all right.

Plagued as he was with severe headaches he reached only as far as Kamloops the first day, Calgary the second, Regina the third. Finding Stacey's nightmares not as severe when she slept during daylight hours they drove only at night, refuelling by gas jugs stored in the trunk. Near dawn Richard would pull off the Trans-Canada onto a side-road and scout out a shaded and well-concealed spot to sleep. To conserve what little money he had left they camped in a musty old canvas tent, one that had belonged to Richard's father.

The kilometres ticked off rapidly until they came to Ontario.

There Richard's Buick began having troubles, and troubles he couldn't immediately diagnose. About 2:00 a.m. on their sixth night the car finally quit altogether, and he and Stacey wound up at a twenty-four hour truck stop. It was one on Highway 11 near North Bay. It was also one Sally Stanton stopped at for coffee that workday morning on her way back to Muskoka.

Overhearing a very bedraggled Richard make desperate inquires with another patron about how to deal with his car problems, Sally was not long in offering help. "We'll tow the car to my place with the one-ton and you can work on it there," she eventually said, motioning to her landscaping truck. "If fixing it takes days, then it takes days. I'll put you up." Richard had no idea what to make of this seemingly overgenerous offer, but he was desperate, and with Stacey half-asleep in his arms he accepted.

Richard needed a long, frustrating week to fix his car. Although during this time Sally didn't ask many questions, he often noticed her eyes on him, and they were worried eyes. Perhaps it was Richard seeming a little too anxious to be on his way, or perhaps his haggard appearance and nervous manner. Regardless, somehow this woman knew he had more than car troubles, and that in turn made Richard uncomfortable. He simply wanted to get back on the road and forever solve his and Stacey's problems. He saw absolutely no sense in trying to explain.

With Sally's North Bay job completed early she was off work for this week. Since Richard was consumed with the car, most of her time she graciously spent with Stacey. Together the two swam in the river, played board games inside, and baked. They got along very well, Richard noticed, and on the Friday of that week he also noticed something else: Stacey slept through the entire night. So routinely had he been up with her each evening the previous months that he now woke on his own, but on Friday it was only to find Stacey fast asleep. Before he had recovered from this first surprise, however, there came another. The following Saturday afternoon he emerged from under the Buick to find a note tucked behind a windshield wiper. It was written in Stacey's large, printed letters, and decorated with tiny musical notes.

We found a house by a river,
Where we ate, funned, and slept.
The lady said we could stay for'iver,
And that's an offer I hereby accept.

Looking up Richard scanned the lot and house, and soon spotted Stacey. She was seated beside Sally at her piano, and was smiling brightly through the window.

So, for the time being at least, the part of Richard that loved his daughter — and this was his only part — decided they would stay. In September he entered Stacey into school, landed a job as a mechanic, and, slowly but surely, there grew some semblance of normality again to their lives. First months, then years passed without their resuming their eastward journey. And although many opportunities arose for them to move into their own residence, somehow Sally always persuaded them to stay. Stanton Corner was now their 'retirement home' as much as hers, she contended, yet never explained. She really didn't need to.

Joel Thompson was only several months in the world when Sally Stanton left home for good on that chilly day in November, 1972. Born also into quite a different family than Sally's — lower working class and very liberal — you would think the two had nothing in common. Yet Joel's fate in life was perhaps also sealed from the beginning. As his somewhat simple grandfather contended, not a great deal grows on a stone.

Tina Thompson never bothered asking the last name of an out-of-town stranger she picked up at an Ottawa bar in January of '72. When later learning she was pregnant she therefore was left fending for herself. And although also unemployed, addicted to bar hopping, and greatly discouraged by her elderly, widowed father, she had the baby and did not even consider adoption. Much like someone buying a dog to garner attention she secretly believed having a baby would make her a veritable star among her bar friends. She'd be doing something "serious", and would be an all-knowing authority on mothering from behind her cigarette smoke and beer.

The first four years of Joel's life, predictably, were a disaster. Tina proved a worse mother than her father even feared, staying out to all hours of the night, and when at home often ignoring her baby for lengthy periods. She did indeed achieve her desired celebrity status as a new mother, but after about a year it faded, and Joel then only became "a major pain in the ass." Her father, already in his seventies, could do little to alleviate this problem, simply not having the steam for parenting anymore. Also, what meagre help he could offer ended just after Joel's fourth birthday when, yelling for the boy to return home, he died suddenly of a heart attack. This left Tina utterly on her own, and her next move surprised no one.

Tina's cousin, Barry Olsen, lived with his wife Maureen in a modest house ten miles outside Ottawa. The couple was childless, and by choice. From their beginnings they declared themselves unfit for parenting. But, after considerable pleading by Tina, and her insisting she would provide child support, they did finally agree to take Joel. Tina delivered him, along with his few clothes and toys, on a Saturday in June. Leaving she all but spun gravel in her father's car. That night she would go on six-bar, 'home from the war' spree, leaving her teary-eyed with joy and bedded with a passing railway worker.

In the six years following, however, Joel's childhood became as close to normal as it ever would. As they suggested, Barry and Maureen were by no means perfect guardians, but through a determined effort they did a decent job caring for the boy. Barry even took Joel camping several times, and Maureen made sure Christmas and birthdays were special occasions. In light of this Joel became quite attached to the couple, even referring to them as 'mother' and 'father' at times. But that, naturally, only made what happened next all the tougher.

As much as Barry and Maureen wanted to keep Joel, in time they simply couldn't afford to. Tina, predictably, had never come through with her promised child support, and as Joel grew so did his upkeep. The final blow, however, was Maureen getting laid off. The Olsens were already barely making ends meet, and so, they insisted, Tina would have to again assume responsibility for her child. And this time they were unmovable.

Joel's chin all but dragged on the ground the October day Tina came to get him. What followed would also do nothing to lift it. 'Family' activities changed to keeping track of who at his grandfather's now ramshackle house was drinking what, and tidying the basement when only one guest and Tina remained. But not shockingly, within a year he would have to forego such joys.

Joel, now eleven, was next shipped to an uncle of Tina's. Like Barry and Maureen, Harvey Aston also lived just outside Ottawa. Unlike the couple, however, Harvey, a surly, temperamental man in his late fifties, made it clear to Tina her son would have to earn his keep.

For the next several years Joel became virtually a slave to his latest guardian. From splitting firewood to shovelling snow to housework he was rarely without an assigned chore. Despite aiming to please and working hard, however, neither the quality nor quantity of his work ever sufficed. Often during the evening Harvey, losing his temper, would slap Joel around for his "laziness" and several times the boy sustained cuts and bruises. All came to a head, though, late one Friday evening in June of 1985. Soon after arriving home from work Harvey flew into a particularly bad rage, and this time Joel fled. He easily outran the older man and was soon well away, and for good.

His first instinct that night told him to return to Barry and Maureen. When he did, however, walking almost fifteen miles in a cool rain, he found the house now had new owners. They also were not especially appreciative of having their door banged on in the middle of the night. Soaked to the bone, and starting out at nearly 3:00 a.m., he walked another twelve miles to the only other place available to him.

For two weeks Joel slept in his grandfather's garage, hidden behind spider-infested planter boxes stored on a high shelf. About seven in the evening each day, when Tina left for the bars, he would slip through a back window of the house and carefully pilfer food, making sure to not take overly noticeable amounts. For those several weeks he was successful at this, too, until, out of agonizing hunger, he swiped an entire loaf of bread. Footprints were also subsequently noticed, ones Tina even recognized, and when the police pulled into the driveway Joel was not long in making the prints lead into the bush behind the house.

For five years Joel did not have a home. Drifting endlessly he slept anywhere he could find that was tolerable, or sometimes not — from barns to abandoned cars to the cramped nooks under apartment stairs. He also was forced to essentially eat anything he could find. When having no success panhandling he would climb into grocery store dumpsters just after dawn to search out discarded breads, cakes, and vegetables, eating many that had molded. Sometimes these made him vomit, but out of sheer hunger, within an hour he would be rummaging again, often frantically. And so years of his life passed.

It was in the fall of 1989 than Joel began writing letters home. With a pencil and bits of paper he found on roadsides he would write long, detailed accounts of his glorious adventures. These he would drop in mail boxes whenever he encountered them. He pictured a smiling mother, father, and other family reading the letters, inspired at times, saddened others. Their beloved Joel was living life to the fullest, but they missed him dearly, longed for the day he would return home. There would be a great celebration then; he'd be smothered in hugs and gifts, and for hours his dear mother would hold him tightly, and sob in relief.

Amidst writing such letters he though often of home. So clear were his memories of family members he could even have any of them join him in his adventures for a time. Whenever he came upon anything especially interesting, for example — like a car wreck or a fast motorcycle — he would talk it over with his brother. He could even picture his elder sibling's expressions, could watch him light a cigarette as he spoke. He also had many a conversation about his future with his father. His senior had all sorts of ideas regarding what career his talented son might adopt — he might be a fireman, a race car driver, or even an NHL hockey player. Best of all, however, he enjoyed the games he would play with his little sister. Their favourite was 'Pop Can Kick', scored by how many kicks each managed. Many a night they spent zigzagging down roads, jostling one another to score the next kick. One might even break the record.

It was during one such late-night match that a badly-rusting car pulled to the side of the road just ahead of him. Sweating and breathing heavily from the game, he opened the creaky passenger door and got in without a word.

"Where are you headed?" a husky, dimly-lit driver asked, pulling back onto the road.

"Headed?" Joel brought filthy hands to a scarred and equally dirty face.

"Where are you going?"

Several seconds of silence, then, "Next town."

"Is that where you live?"

"Need to send a letter home. My parents are waitin' for it. Maybe Grandma too."

Through a stench that by this time had filled the car, the driver said, "And where's home?"

"In the next town." Joel suddenly turned to look out his window.

"What?"

"Thought I saw something."

"Really? What did you see?"

"My dog, I think. Might ... have been my brother or something, though."

The driver again glanced at Joel a moment, then resumed watching the road. "How long have you been travelling?"

"How long? My hair's not long."

The driver considered questioning further, but ultimately left it at that.

The following morning Joel woke to the rocking of several sacks of grass seed being unloaded from the aging Buick's rear seat, and when looking back he saw Sally Stanton smiling at him.

So began life for Joel Thompson at Stanton Corner. With Richard's help Sally established a modest room for him in the attic, and through the yard-sale circuit each Saturday they gradually bought furnishings. The room wasn't much, but it was his, and he came to take great pride in it. Sally never needed to clean or even tidy the room.

Despite becoming quite settled in, Joel continued writing letters home. These he would present to Sally at breakfast, and always she would promise to mail them. Each time, also, she wound up wiping a tear from her eye. The letters were never more than indiscernible scratchings, explanations, apologies, or promises to family he would, she knew, never see again. But they seemed extremely important to Joel and so she never questioned them. She also never asked questions after watching Joel play various games in the yard, seemingly with an imaginary friend. Or after times he stood almost motionless for hours down at the edge of the river, seemingly talking at length either with himself, or with those he dearly missed.

In the years following Sally would welcome other 'retirees' to Stanton Corner, some staying merely weeks, some years. Megan and Paul Howard found a home here, and so too, for a time, Dave Brooks and Glenna Case. Like their predecessors they were the depressed and the confused and the broken, and for each Sally Stanton became a saviour.

None could agree when The Corner's singing tradition began. Some claimed it arose at a birthday party, others that it started with several residents joining Sally at the piano one afternoon, more gradually joining during future sessions. Either way, at some point Sally opened her sizable repertoire of songs to other voices, and at least twice a week those voices could be heard up and down the river. In a sense the composer's music did remain private, however; never did the group perform outside the house. Some who paddled the river may have considered they were practicing for an

upcoming event, but this was never the case. The music, whether
consciously recognized as such, was solely a means of personal
healing, a medicinal ritual in lives gone awry.

It was Joel Thompson who stumbled upon a certain homemade
plaque one morning in August of 1995. Almost entirely grown over
in tall grass, it was mostly rotted, and in stumbling Joel broke it in
two. When he brought the plaque to Richard Hastings' attention,
however, the elder resident was not long in piecing it together and
deciphering the crudely-routered letters. He was also not long in
forming a plan.

Fearing someone, meaning Joel, might accidentally say
something to Sally, he kept Stanton Corner's tenth anniversary
party a secret until only about a week beforehand. Then, informing
all those who lived or had lived at The Corner, he organized an
event befitting the occasion.

As things went, it almost didn't happen. The Friday of the party
Sally's truck broke down on the highway, and for hours none
waiting at the house knew of her whereabouts. At last, however, she
arrived home, and proceeded to almost fall down so loud was the
'Surprise!" she received. Fourteen-year-old Stacey Hastings was the
ring leader in this regard.

What followed was the gift of the maple armchair, songs with
Sally at the piano, supper, and a cake with 'Stanton Corner' joining
ten candles. Lastly, soon after presenting Sally with the cake Glenna
Case seated herself at the piano. The others quickly took their
places around it, and their short song, the last of the evening, was of
their own creation:

We sing
Of a special and lasting place.
Our home, our salvation.
A place granted as a gift,
A place where life's waters run slower,
And more peaceful yet.
For this we ever give thanks
Our precious bend in the river.

With that Sally Stanton gazed again toward the front window, to where she'd earlier spent several minutes solemnly pondering her beginnings. In turn she now thought of the unfoldings of her last ten years, of the lives she'd touched and been touched by, of hope for society's future. And taking a deep breath, she blew out her candles, and smiled.

3

LETTERS TO BRENNAN LAKE

Fred Sutton, seated wearing a faded bathrobe, gazed through the large picture window of his daughter's cottage, scowling. What a pathetic waste, he yet again mused. The bums didn't even deserve the place.

Turning toward a back bedroom he grumbled, "The bums don't even deserve the place, you know that?"

His daughter, dressed in a gray skirt and white blouse, entered the living room spraying blonde, freshly-styled hair. "I know they don't, Dad. But why let it bother you so much? Lots of people in this world don't deserve everything they have." Stopping beside her father's chair she offered a goofy smile. "Like me, for instance."

"They never use the place," Fred continued undaunted while Christina kissed his wrinkled forehead, "and meanwhile it goes to complete rot. My own son-in-law even has to cut their grass just so we don't have to look at an overgrown lawn." He stabbed at the window with a thick, worn finger. "Now that's not right."

Christina, moving toward the side door, said, "Bryan really doesn't mind, Dad. It's not a large lawn, and ... they're paying him well."

Fred huffed. "It's big enough. And it looks like someone put a fair effort into landscaping that lot, all to have it go to waste."

"I'm sure someone put a ton of work into the place. But why worry so much? Why let it ruin your summer? You're here to relax."

"Maybe it bothers me because I don't have anything else to do but let it bother me. How come I have nothing to do?"

Christina sat on a bench near the door and began slipping dress shoes onto her nyloned feet. Tiredly she said, "Because, as I mentioned, you're here for the summer to take it easy. Why don't you start another novel? Or work in the garden today — you enjoy that."

"I'm sick of the garden. Besides, seems like those wildflowers growing up in it look better than your store-bought ones anyway. You should open your eyes to these things. You keep yourself so busy with office stuff I swear this place passes you by."

To this Fred's back received a grin, and Christina rose from the bench. "Yes, Dad, I suppose it does. So why don't you get dressed and go out for a walk and see all those nice things while I head to work. Com'on now — it's a beautiful morning, a perfect start to the week."

"I've a good mind to make some phone calls."

"Don't be silly. Just leave things be."

Once more Fred huffed, and as Christina soon headed to her car he again grumbled, "Bums don't even deserve the place."

As his daughter suggested, it truly was a fine Monday morning Fred Sutton soon stepped into. The day was bright and warm and the breeze drifting off the lake carried the fresh scent of the west-shore pines. Above, in the deep blue of the sky, he even noticed a rare eagle doing slow, graceful circles. Indeed the morning seemed scarcely improvable, one that, as Fred was becoming fond of saying to himself, "made you withdraw any and all complaints from the head honcho." Curiously, since arriving at the lake in early June he had seen many such days, but not until recently, in late July, did he begin appreciating them. He mused over this as he began walking the grassy shore of the lake, purposefully.

Brennan Lake was tiny but neatly tucked into the heart of Muskoka. It was shaped like an acorn, its cottagers liked to say, with

most having built along the 'crown'. The one exception was a green
bungalow nestled among pines at the tip of the 'cup', the western
end of the lake.

It was, to Fred's taste, quite a fine-looking cottage: small but
sufficient, stylish but not overdone, "the sort of place a guy could
really enjoy." And therefore a terrible thing to waste.

Since arriving at the lake for the summer he had yet to see
anyone at the west-shore cottage. If this was someone's little
getaway they certainly were not getting away much. You would,
Fred thought, at least lend the place to friends if for whatever
reason you couldn't make it up from the city, or from wherever you
lived. To leave any cottage idle in the summer seemed to him, lately
at least, almost sacrilegious.

Spurred by such an annoyance, and surely a touch of boredom,
as the summer progressed Fred found himself walking the lake's
shore on weekdays while his daughter worked, and in the midst,
poking about the abandoned cottage. He became, for reasons he
could not exactly pin down, consumed with gaining an answer to
the owners' mysterious absence. Were they too busy? Had they lost
interest in the place? He wanted to know, needed to know. If
somehow he received a satisfactory answer to this question, one
excusing the owners for their cottage crimes, he would no longer be
bothered, and so could get on with enjoying his summer. He could,
that is, get on with relaxing, just as his daughter suggested.

He gained scant insight into this mystery from exploring the
yard. The small, overgrown garden, the tiny dock with its
overturned canoe, the rain-smoothed driveway — none of these
offered any clues. Only about a week passed, therefore, before his
hunger led him to window-peeking, and to what naturally came
next.

He had little trouble finding a key, 'hidden' as it was in such a
ridiculously obvious spot — on top of a porch lamp. He also had
little trouble justifying his uninvited visit; if the owners were leaving
the cottage unattended, then heck, he was doing them a favour.
What if, for instance, the roof were leaking? A summer's worth of
rain could do serious damage.

The cottage proved to have a main room, a kitchen, a tiny bathroom, and three bedrooms in back. The layout, similar to his daughter's cottage, was typical, but to Fred typical for a good reason: it worked. The living room hosted an assortment of modest and well-worn furniture, and wall shelves held equally aged-looking wood carvings, knickknacks, and framed photographs. One photo Fred examined showed two kids, a girl and slightly younger boy, together with a frail woman whose brown hair and sharp features made her obviously the children's mother. Seated on the cottage's dock with her legs in the water, she was watching the kids swim. All wore genuine smiles, Fred noted, but the badly-faded picture was clearly taken quite some time ago.

For the first several visits Fred only randomly poked about the front rooms. Once again, however, a lack of evidence pushed him further, and this meant having a look at the bedrooms. The northernmost was the smallest of the three, and by its bright colours and storybook mural on one wall he surmised it belonged to the kids in the living room photo. The middle bedroom was bigger but lacked personal effects, and he gathered this was intended for guests. The last room was the largest, boasting a queen-sized bed and a walk-in closet. It also contained a long, clearly homemade dresser of rough maple, however, and it was on this rustic piece of furniture Fred made his most enlightening discovery.

Like the dresser, a small wooden box resting on it also seemed homemade but was better-crafted, even sporting dovetail corners. The box lacked a lid, however — or if one existed it was not in sight — and thus while scanning the room from the door Fred easily noticed what lay inside the box: letters, dozens of them.

Yes, it was terribly wrong of him to do so, he knew, but on the very day he discovered the letters Fred Sutton began reading them. Naturally he never mentioned his newfound pastime to Christina, nor even his visiting the west-shore cottage; she would surely have a fit, and a justified one. But somehow he simply could not help himself. Terrifically bored at this early point in the summer, he felt the letters possibly held the answer to the mystery of the absentee cottagers, the only thing at the lake presently interesting him.

And so he began reading, turning over the pile of letters to begin with the most dated first, as was his style tackling virtually anything. "You start from the beginning and work your way to the end," he often lectured to Christina. Besides, he had a whole summer to spare.

The letters he persevered in reading over the first several weeks were short and, as with the exterior of the cottage, offered Fred few insights. Reminders of upcoming events, recipes, construction details — more like notes, he reflected. Not until the third Monday in July, indeed this very morning he saw the eagle, did he come to a longer letter offering more substance. Like those previous, the papers were yellowed but still readable. So soon after rounding the lake's west bay and entering the cottage, Fred started into it. He read very slowly, the best he could manage nowadays, relaxing his terribly nosy and uninvited self on a bed he found quite comfortable.

September 16, 1967

Dear Mindy,

So glad there are such things in this world as cottages! I know Jamie insists there's still a great deal of work left on your new Muskoka treasure, but the place seemed just dandy to us — may you enjoy it for many years to come!

I simply had to write and thank you again, dear cousin, for providing us with such a wonderful time this summer. Howard, little Nancy, and I had a delightful week, and you, Jamie, and the kids could not have been better hosts. Between swimming, sunbathing, canoeing, walks, games, and chats out under the stars we had a superb holiday. One thing I must comment on in particular was our meals! It really is true food tastes better outdoors, especially in the country. When I think of the barbecues we had my mouth starts watering instantly. And the way we were so limited in what we could prepare, lacking so many modern conveniences, a little extra flavouring at times never hurt. How we howled when Jamie bit into that hamburger after Shelley and Nancy had rolled the patty along the beach several times! Ah, but this is the sort of fun that makes cottaging the joy it is, isn't it? If only we could convince poor Jamie!

For his part, Howard seems to have quite enjoyed helping your husband attend to various cottage chores, and batting around ideas for future improvements. He has hardly hushed about this since returning home. Oh the effort a cottage takes! Listening to Jamie we certainly came to better understand the work that's involved, and if he intended a hint we've taken it! We will continue being more than happy to help out with whatever needs doing, from the lake garden (as your dear husband calls it) to the footings to cleaning inside. We will help in any way we can; we so much want you and Jamie to enjoy your cottage, not be a slave to it. As for Shelley and Nicky, what needs saying other than they are truly in their element in Muskoka, and it would be such a tragedy if their fun was in any way hindered. We feel this especially applies to Nicky. He is so much like his father, so looks up to him, and we hope Jamie's bothers about the cottage don't grow to the point they become contagious. For both your kids, may their cottage memories have a glow about them!

While I'm on this topic of projects, as your elder I must remind you to take care when walking down to the lake, Mindy. I know you feel quite giddy and daring at the cottage, especially when you first arrive, but rock-infested Muskoka was not made for fragile legs the likes of yours. Jamie tells me he intends to build stone steps here and there along the walkway to make things safer for you, but as I've mentioned, with all the other projects he insists must be done it may be a while before you have those steps. Please do be careful.

I don't believe I told you but on the Thursday of our week, when you, Jamie, and the three kids were in town, Howard and I took a stroll down to the falls at the end of your road. What are they called again? Sasha Falls? We had only driven previously and my how much more you experience when you walk! The falls proved almost boring in the scope of this sunny afternoon, so many interesting cottagers did we speak with. Everyone was unbelievably friendly and inviting. On both the way to the falls and on the way back we were invited in for drinks. Although we declined, the second couple — the Mitchells — even offered us a full lunch! It was so different from the strolls we take in the city. I don't know why it is, but urban people, as all these cottagers were, become much friendlier

*when they're out of the city. Maybe it's a matter of less stress after escaping
the city's hustle and bustle, or being near wild things, or perhaps something
else. I really don't have the answer. But it makes Howard and I sad not
being able to afford a cottage of our own, wondering how much friendlier
we ourselves might be.*

*Anyway, in closing, thanks again for treating us to such a wonderful
week this summer, Mindy, and for tolerating us. We will surely accept your
invitation for another visit next year, and we look forward to that
immensely. Howard, in fact, is already making a rather lengthy checklist
of activities!*

Love,

Gwendolyn

Over the remainder of that week Fred read yet more of the
letters, gradually working his way through the thick pile. Most of
these succeeding writings again proved quite short, but together
with those lengthier they summarized cottage events over almost
the next twenty years. Most notably, during the summer of 1971
Shelley and Nicky sampled some poisonous berries growing behind
the cottage and landed in the hospital. Thereafter a paranoid father
greatly hindered their freedom. Three years later a major
thunderstorm brought down an old birch. It severely damaged the
northeast corner of the cottage, and once again Jamie was
consumed. But mixed with such unfortunate events were countless
pleasant occasions which in her letters cousin Gwendolyn,
seemingly visiting every year with her family, was more than happy
to reflect upon. In the end, therefore, Fred could not yet see any
reason for the cottage now remaining empty; the positives the place
offered seemed to outweigh the negatives.

On Friday his son-in-law arrived, as usual, from Toronto for
the weekend. Bryan was a bank manager, and unlike Christina, a
bookkeeper, was not able to relocate his work to Muskoka for the
summer. Every weekend, however, he drove up to the cottage,

arriving late afternoon.

Fred was not long in questioning him about the west-shore cottage, drawing his son-in-law onto the front deck after their Friday supper, which Christina always insisted on making a special occasion.

"So what did they say when they hired you to cut the lawn?"

Bryan, still adjusting the "down-home duds" he had replaced his suit with upon arrival, stared at Fred a moment before answering, "Just that they'd be away for the summer, Dad."

"Nothing else?"

"Nothing else. And it really doesn't bother me about looking after their lawn, if that's what you're getting at. They paid me well."

"Bloody well better have. You're supposed to be up here getting away from that bank and taking a break, not working."

"I realize. But then, pardon me for saying so — you are too. Christina especially feels that way. She says you've earned it."

Fred turned. "Earned it? What have I done to earn it? She won't let me do any work."

"I know, but she's thinking of ... older times."

"What older times? You two have only had this place a few years, and this is my first visit. And I just got here in June, for God's sake."

"I meant older times as when she was growing up. All the great memories you made for her. She's told me a lot of stories."

"Probably overdid it," Fred whispered, and remained silent a moment, looking strained. At last he said, "So anyone ever come around when you've been over there."

Bryan wearily ruffled his once office-neat black hair. "Nope. Why?"

Fred's eyes widened. "Why? Because I'd like to give them a talking to, that's *why*. They've got some nerve letting a nice cottage like that go to waste. There should be laws against it. Did they mention anything about having run into problems, or that they intended to sell the place?"

"No. But how come you're asking? Thinking of buying it?" Bryan grinned, slyly.

Fred again turned in his chair, glaring. "Make fun of the notion all you want, Smarty. Strikes me as a heck of good little place. A guy could do worse."

His grin slowly disappearing, Bryan said in a sincere tone, and softly, "Yes, I'd say that cottage is right down your alley, Dad. This whole lake, actually. You seem to be starting to enjoy yourself, I've noticed, and I'm glad."

"The lake ... has its merits, I suppose."

"So then why let that place down at the far end bother you so much? Just take it easy."

"We'll see about that," was Fred's stern answer, and this time it was his son-in-law's turn to look strained.

The following Monday, soon after Christina left for work, Fred resumed his letter-reading. The morning was gray and drizzly and he saw little else to do anyway. He was surprised, however, by how much he enjoyed the walk around the lake; the glistening tree leaves, the earthy scent of the water, the soothing patter of the light rain. It was so fresh. "I'll take a rainy day at the cottage over a sunny day in the city anytime," he had once heard Bryan say, and he was now inclined to agree.

He again saw no sign of anyone having been in the green cottage, and was cavalier about entering. After drawing the next collection of stapled pages from the overturned pile in the letter box he lay on the bed and began reading, slowly as usual. He was now about halfway through the pile.

July 6, 1984

Dear Mindy,

Just thought I'd drop you a note. You were wondering about Nancy and I'm pleased to report she landed the job out west. We now therefore have an empty nest! Where have all the years gone? It seems like yesterday Nancy, Shelley, and Nicky were kids and now, along with all of them graduating from school and leaving home, Shelley is married. We're getting old, Mindy. Might be time to break out the canes.

The wedding was fantastic! Such perfect weather, and I think holding it at the cottage was a terrific idea. The pictures you sent were marvellous. We particularly enjoyed the one with the bride and groom down by the shore of the lake, and the one with Jamie pretending to be on the verge of tossing his new son-in-law in that same lake (or was he pretending?!) Howard and I are going to frame those two and put them in the living room with our raft of other cottage pictures. You've provided us with quite a collection over the years.

We were so sorry to hear about Jamie's accident, especially considering the timing, only a few weeks after such a fine wedding. Who would have guessed that beam under the cottage could have rotted that badly? I hope his arm heals well; what a fright the whole incident must have given him. I'd have nightmares for years, myself. I hope, too, the cost of the repairs was not high. As I told you by phone, Howard and I insist on contributing our share to 'The Cottage Fund'. We feel you were wise in having that contractor fix the foundation right away; I'm sure the longer poor Jamie helplessly looked at it wearing a cast the more uptight he would have become.

We received your invite for an August visit and we'd be delighted. Considering recent events, we've resolved to do anything and everything that needs doing around the cottage to keep Jamie content. I hope you don't mind me saying so, but how he frets over the place now! Howard and I have certainly learned over the years when to stay clear. Sadly, that back corner of the cottage collapsing is not likely to improve Jamie's cheer, nor Nicky's. I fear you may be right when you said he's stepping into his father's shoes in a certain respect — how he can grumble about the cottage himself! Howard tells me he's working on a cure; he's going to get Nicky doing more fun things this summer and not let him worry about cottage chores so much. Like taking him rock-climbing, if his mother's heart can stand it. What fun Howard had doing this as a kid, and he wants to pass his skills on. Hope Nicky proves a willing student.

I must tell you again — Howard and I absolutely loved the special gifts you sent us at Christmas this year. We had no idea when we got the kids making those crafts that rainy afternoon so many summers back that we'd ultimately be the recipients. We will treasure these items forever. We've put Shelley's pressed fern collages above the fireplace and Nicky's driftwood statues (or soldiers, as he called them) in the kitchen, keeping

guard over the refrigerator. I can't imagine you giving us lovelier
Christmas gifts, Mindy. Be sure to thank the kids again for us.

As a final note, please don't plan anything exceptional for us like you
did last year with the party. We very much appreciate the thought, but the
cottage on its own is special enough, and you know Jamie's not up to much
this summer. Let's give the poor guy a break.

Love,

Gwendolyn

On a Friday in mid-August Christina and Bryan started their
two-week summer holiday. With both present during the day Fred's
letter-reading temporarily ceased, and how. "I've up for everything,
Dad!" Christina said in a bubbly, joking tone when she arrived
home from her last day of work, but Fred soon realized she was not
kidding. In the days following she, along with Bryan, drew him into
every cottage pastime imaginable. During mornings the three
usually went for walks on the main road or for hikes through the
neighbouring woods. Afternoons they often spent swimming, and
evenings brought barbecues, guests, and cards. Cottage chores were
very much kept in the background, Fred noticed, with his kids
insisting they do only what was absolutely necessary. "A cottage
doesn't need to be a perfect thing," Bryan, most notably, said to him
one afternoon, and he soon came to agree. This Jamie he'd been
reading about had it all wrong; you went to a cottage to first and
foremost take it easy and enjoy what the cottage setting had to offer.
Else what was the point. It became to him all so obvious.

"Ever really take a look at the lake?" he asked his daughter from
his dock chair early on one of her holiday afternoons, and soon after
she arrived for a swim.

Playfully kicking off her sandals she answered, "Excuse me?"

"I said, have you ever really looked at the lake? Really studied it?"

Christina shrugged. "I've been around Brennan long enough to
know it, I think."

"But have you ever taken an hour or two and just stared into the water and watched everything that went on? The fish, the frogs, the water spiders, the drifting bits of wood and plant, and so on?"

Christina smiled, approaching her still-bathrobed father and running her fingers through his silvery hair, which stood up in places. "You've had yourself quite a morning."

"Scoff all you want. I've found the lake very interesting. You might too."

"I'm not scoffing, Dad. I'm just ... surprised." After moving to the edge of the dock she turned and added, "Surprised in a nice way, though."

"Why would you be so surprised?"

But to this Fred received no reply, his daughter evidently deciding she should now dive in.

Evenings became Fred's most treasured time during his kids' holidays. After supper he invariably sat with Christina and Bryan on the front deck, watching the sun make its slow decent toward the western shore. Sometimes the three talked about the day's events, but often they simply sat, silently relishing. Fred loved how shiny and smooth the lake became during the evening, and how the trees and grasses were so richly greened in the dimming light. The sounds he also came to cherish; the croaking frogs, the occasional laughter from neighbouring cottages, and especially, the cracklings of a bonfire. Usually someone on the lake each night lit one near shore, and he loved watching excited kids play around it and roast marshmallows. Even from a distance he could see their smiling faces, brightened in flashes by the flames, and couldn't help smiling himself. And beyond all this was the smell of wood smoke drifting across the lake, blending with the ever-present scent of those west-shore pines.

Such times made for the best summer Fred could imagine, and he came to dread the approaching day when the season ended and Christina took him back to the city. He even began secretly marking the remaining days off on a calendar, much as he might have done as a boy. Perhaps this was only fitting, too, for at this point in the summer he felt like a boy again — reinvigorated and refreshed and renewed. He thus very much regretted not having spent more time in cottage country in previous years. If only he had realized.

"I know now why they never come around."

It was a Saturday morning, about a week after Christina and Bryan finished their holidays, and only several days before father and daughter were to pack up and return to the city. Fred had just sat down to breakfast at the kitchen table.

In the midst of pouring his coffee, Christina said, "Why who never comes around, Dad?"

Fred pointed with his cereal spoon to the window, to the west end of the lake. "Why *they* don't. I've figured it out."

His daughter glanced at the green cottage, then with a shaky voice said, "Okay. Why don't they?"

Fred squinted at her. "Death in the family, and they haven't regrouped yet. Who knows, too, whether they ever will."

Christina, slowly seating herself, said, "I see. And how, might I ask, did you surmise all that?"

Fred's eyes sparkled. "Oh, let's just say I sorted things out. But never mind how. Let's look at the bright side. Now I can forgive them for wasting the cottage and put it all behind me. Like you wanted me to — remember?"

"Yes, I do," Christina answered in almost a whisper, her gaze turning again to the west shore. "I suppose it's a good thing you know what's what."

She drove over, such that her father could not see her destination, telling him they needed a few groceries from town. The laneway leading into the little green cottage began just after the lake's west end, and she followed it slowly, minding the rough patches that, it saddened her to see, had multiplied so quickly.

Her first clue came soon after arriving. Upon retrieving the key and entering the cottage she immediately noticed familiar footprints on the door mat. Yes, he'd been in, she alarmingly thought to herself, and what on earth did he find?

She searched the cottage, calmly at first, then almost frantically, cursing herself for not having hidden the door key in a different spot. She noticed nothing out of place in the front rooms, however; either her father had not looked at much or had been very careful.

Soon, though, she turned her attention to the bedrooms, and it was in the largest she at last saw more signs of someone having been in. At first it was the slightly-wrinkled bedspread. Then she noticed the box on the dresser, and in particular, the crudely-folded topmost letter.

Nervously grasping the hand-written pages, and seating herself on the bed much as her father had done, Christina began reading, all the while wondering.

June 16, 1997

Dear Shelley,

We've just returned from Florida and I felt like writing you. Hope everyone in your family is doing well, especially your father. We do wish him a fine summer — he so deserves it after all that's happened.

I trust you received the pictures of your mother I sent you several weeks ago (we had prints made for ourselves to keep, so don't worry about returning them). Howard and I thought you would appreciate this little collection. They span a great many years, and we feel bring out the wonderful qualities your dear mother had — her generosity, playfulness, and compassion for others. I can not possibly describe to you how much we miss her. Anytime Howard and I speak of her at length these days I invariably have myself a cry and my poor husband suddenly needs to do an errand. We loved Mindy so much, Shelley.

Your brother wrote and informed us your parents' legal matters have been tidied up, and now all your father has to do is get better, and we're hopeful he will. Howard and I dream of the day we can speak to the 'old' Jamie again. Even though he's still the same basic person, it's tragic when you can't share memories, especially those associated with your mother and the cottage. But we've taken the liberty of speaking with several psychologists (I hope you don't mind) and we do understand the reality of the situation, that your father may never recover. Such a shock that horrible accident at the cottage gave him! He, like everyone, knew how weak in the legs Mindy was, but it must still have been a terrifying surprise to see her take a fall like that. And to lose someone you so dearly loved, to see her life end so abruptly, so close, with your very eyes. It really is no wonder your father has lost all memory of your mother and the cottage, and so many things and people he associated with her. The professionals can offer their clinical explanations about why Jamie can remember some things but not others. To us, however, his predicament boils down to one thing: his deep and lasting love for dear Mindy.

But — I'm so sorry — on to brighter things.

The cottage! Oh, the memories! The mornings, the afternoons, the evenings — what delights we shared. Anytime I close my eyes I can be there. Anyone who knows such experiences also knows they can never be given value; they're priceless and precious and to be treasured forever.

Through the cottage, to begin, we have watched you and your brother, and our Nancy, enjoy some of the best times of your lives. How you kids loved to swim and splash in the shallows! I sometimes wondered whether the three of you would grow fins. And how you also loved the games we would play, and staying up late, and the pillow fights. I could go on forever. It was of no surprise to our family when you announced you were building your own cottage on the lake. We can't imagine you being happier anywhere else, and we're sure Nicky (when he settles down a bit!) will also one day have a summer cabin. He has not shown much interest in cottaging over the last five years or so, we realize, but we believe that will change, or at least we hope so. Perhaps, as with all life's experiences, it takes time for the best to rise to the top of the milk jug. Was that silly? As your mother would say, "So be it!"

Regarding that mother — where to start? Never was she more energetic, playful, and downright goofy than she was at the cottage. Remember how, when we arrived, she would charge down to the dock ahead of everyone and jump in the lake? Even with those bad legs of hers you kids could never keep up. And how about that afternoon, when you, Nancy, and Nicky were so little, she dressed up as a clown, and for nearly an hour none of you knew it was her?! Or the way she insisted everyone, when at the cottage, be referred to by their middle names? She could be so *much fun, and the cottage brought out that side of her like nowhere else.*

Last, but surely not least, we have such pleasant memories of your father at the cottage. I admit he could be edgy about the place, what with it being so much work, but we truly enjoyed him nonetheless, and we believe in our hearts he also nonetheless truly enjoyed the cottage. Perhaps, if there is a positive side to his memory loss over the accident, it is that he cannot remember the headaches of years past, and thus has a fresh start, a second chance at appreciating the joys of cottaging. And we do hope he does. As I said in the opening of this letter, he so deserves it.

But I should close now; I'm perhaps beginning to ramble, and it's becoming tough to read my handwriting. I am so sorry if this letter upsets you also, but I had such a deep need to share some things with you, Shelley. Please forgive me if this letter only adds to your grief.

Take care, say hello to that fun-loving husband of yours for us, and do extend our best wishes to your father, will you, Dear? If Jamie says, "Who in the heck are Gwendolyn and Howard?" simply tell him we're strangers who wish him well. Our love for him need not be returned.

Best wishes, as always,

Gwendolyn

Carefully folding the letter, Christina placed it back in the wooden box. She then reached under the dresser for the lid. The label on it was embossed, and after placing it on the box she softly ran her fingers over the aged lettering.

Letters To Brennan Lake
The Humble and Beloved Retreat of
Jennifer Melinda and Frederick James
Sutton.

She then made her way out the door, heading to cottage memories still in the making, and to where she knew her dear father would be waiting.

4

HAL'S SAVIOUR

There is, it seems, always a catch to any paradise, and the paradise that is Muskoka is no exception.

When early farming largely failed, owing primarily to poor soils and rocky terrain, tourism took over as the dominant industry. The abundance of picturesque lakes was the district's true treasure, and cottagers along with other visitors soon provided livings, directly or indirectly, for almost all year-round residents. But then came the catch: as much as tourism flourished, it only flourished in the summer. Outside this season, with weather less pleasant and kids attending school, Muskoka's economic roar fell to a whimper. And for most local residents that quieting created a conundrum: how make a living in paradise now?

For the three residents occupying the last lots on Bryant road, the challenge of the off-season was certainly nothing new. Doug Jordan, Ronald Wells, and Harold Scott had lived in Muskoka their entire lives, and within each a feast-and-famine mindset was deeply engrained. Indeed, deeply enough they even guarded it; their homeland's economic reality was the only such reality they had ever known, and so like a religion they defended it staunchly. "Why not just work somewhere else if it's so tough to make a go?" a naive outsider once asked Harold Scott, to which he blared, "Because that, you ass, would be *cheatin'*." And this would have been the answer of any of the three men, the reasonings clear and identical. Muskoka was their home, and unlike the wives they'd all long ago lost, they would stay with it for better or worse.

Doug Jordan's place was the last you came to on Bryant, for here this old and winding country road reached its limit. As the local joke ran, however, it didn't much matter that you'd reached the end of the road because with what you saw here you'd probably stop your car and turn back anyway. If you can picture a 'no-questions' landfill, gravel pit, garage, scrapyard, flea market, produce stand, information bureau, souvenir shop, hunting shop, 'Antique Boutique', and bootleg depot all rolled into two sign-drenched acres, then you may form an adequate image of Doug Jordan's residence. How many entrepreneurial pursuits he had undertaken over the years his two close neighbours were not able to count. Truly, if Ronnie Wells and Hal Scott were ever to see a space shuttle in their neighbour's yard one would likely only shrug and say, "Guess Dougie's doing moon tours this winter." To both the man's imagination and drive simply had no bounds.

But, alas, if the surprising truth must be revealed, ninety-nine out of a hundred of Mr. Jordan's ventures amounted to precious little. Not that he'd ever admit that to you, of course. He had his pride, and a knack for making the uninitiated believe he was only moments away from "going big time" in whatever gem of a product or service any novice expressed interest. Unfortunately, such success was never realized, and indeed, only through the collective rewards of many meagre successes did he even feed his husky frame let alone buy Rolls-Royces. This harsh truth, mind you, never slowed him down. On he went, forever brainstorming ideas, forever prospecting for new minerals in the Muskoka landscape. You could never, as Hal Scott put it, accuse the man of failing to challenge failure.

Frequently coming up short also never hindered Doug Jordan from generously offering his vast talents and business savvy to others. "Money tight these days?" he'd say to a friend. "No problem — have you fixed up in a jiffy." When things went sour, and at card games this was where most Bryant residents placed their money, he would simply concoct another grand scheme to deal with the first. Such helpfulness he especially extended to his dear neighbours, the two men with whom he had shared the 'Zenith of Bryant Road' now close to twenty years. Sharing his gifts with these fine fellows was, as he contended, "simply the right thing to do." And so, when in the winter of 1996 one Harold Scott found himself in a financial predicament, it was only natural Doug Jordan went to his rescue.

The usual messenger delivered the news of Hal's plight. Ronnie Wells lived in a small, ramshackle cabin between Doug Jordan and Harold Scott, and little went on that escaped his restless eyes or wing-like ears. A rickety, jumpy fellow that made you both tired and nervous merely watching him, Ronnie was anywhere and everywhere over the course of an average day. Some Bryant residents questioned whether he even slept. They also questioned whether he was the brightest star in the universe, but not in front of his closest neighbours. Doug Jordan especially defended Ronnie; he was, after all, the mastermind's greatest admirer, what with the fine employment he received from the endless enterprises next door, and Doug much enjoyed being admired. It's nice when someone respects your gifts.

The day Ronnie brought news of Hal was an overcast but relatively mild one in early February. Doug took advantage of this favourable weather to begin building a chicken coop, the foundation of his latest pursuit. Eggs were hot, he declared a week earlier; he would make a killing. He was straightening a scavenged rusty spike when he looked up and saw, behind his roadside lumber display, a red toque bobbing toward him, a little faster than usual.

"What's wrong, Ronnie?" Doug coolly asked when his neighbour reached him.

Ronnie, dressed in a checkered hunting jacket and tattered green vest, stopped short, glancing behind him as though searching for what gave him away.

"I said what's —"

Ronnie's twangy voice at last offered, "Hal's in trouble, Dougie."

Crouched and in the midst of framing the coop's front wall, Doug paused from driving his newly-restored nail. "See a big-build in the paper again?"

"No, it's not that. It's some people. They moved into Hal's basement yesterday while you was away scoutin' for business. And looks like they're stayin' the rest of the damn winter, Dougie."

"Hal invit'em?"

Ronnie shrugged. "He's never said nothin' about people stayin' the winter."

"Never said nothin' to me either. Who are these people?"

"Don' know. The guy, though — Frank — he's a real slick unit. Hair all greased up, and grinnin' behind Hal's back all the time. Also talks to him like he's sellin' him a bridge. And Holly, she looks kinda trampy, I'd say. 'Nough makeup to make a muskrat look pretty."

Doug drove his nail, then said. "They payin' anything?"

"Nope. Ol' slick Frank told me they're not payin' a cent. I don't think they're even helpin' with groceries. Right after they got dropped off Hal went to town and came home with a whole truckload."

Doug stood and stretched his broad back, glancing sternly toward the tidy, gray bungalow next to Ronnie's. "What did Hal have to say about all this?"

"Nothin' much. But you know Hal. Somebody could milk him for every penny and he wouldn't much complain."

Doug nodded; he'd been the recipient of that generosity a few times himself.

Ronnie now delivered the big line, the one he'd rehearsed an hour. In a cold, grave voice he said, "I think Hal's got himself a situation, Dougie."

Knowing full well the implications of this statement, Doug Jordan peered off into space, allowing for the necessary gravity of the request to build. Finally he said, "I *am* busy, though."

Ronnie's eyes bulged. "But ... Hal'll go broke supportin' these two cranks! And you're the only one that can save'im!"

"I suppose," Doug answered modestly, and now having

received the necessary respect he slowly drummed his lower lip with his forefinger. "One thing for damn sure, Ronnie — we couldn't tell Hal anything. You know how shy he's become about accepting my offers of help."

Ronnie nodded. "You'd almost think he was scared of you."

"But, if you're sayin' he really needs me ..." With a grizzled chin Doug motioned to his own house. "The way I see it — if you're havin' hard times you're welcome to move into my house, but you'll be invited in, you sure as hell won't barge in. That'll get you tossed out a window." Waving his hammer menacingly toward Hal's, he said, quietly but gruffly, "Don't worry Ronnie. We'll get rid of the bloody mooches."

Hal Scott was, to most Bryant residents, quite a surprise arrival when he bought his place in 1981. For a good part of his working life he was a developer, and by all appearances very successful. In Muskoka there was a time, in fact, when you'd have been hard-pressed finding what Hal called a "big-build", be it a resort or new subdivision, that didn't have 'Scott Developments' involved. What exactly went wrong no one on Bryant road ever discovered, but things clearly did go wrong, for not long before this articulate, silver-haired businessman bought his modest, end-of-the-road house his company ceased to be. So too did his wife disappear. Some residents speculated he dove too deeply into a bad project, but others simply blamed the usual suspect: the economy. Apparently, they held, developers were every bit as vulnerable to Muskoka's economic duality as anyone. Who was right no one knew for sure, because Hal almost never spoke of his downfall. "Oh, if the moons had been aligned more in my favour ... " was one rare comment, mumbled one night while drinking with his two closest neighbours. When pressed for more details, however, he remained silent, and Doug respectfully resigned. Like himself, he considered, great businessmen were entitled to lick their wounds in private.

Over the years he was blessed with Doug Jordan as a neighbour Hal pretty much kept his distance, business-wise at least. Sure there were social visits; either was always welcome in the other's home.

But he had now politely turned down enough investment opportunities that Doug rarely bothered him anymore. To Hal the man's energy and imagination in making a Muskoka living could be interesting and even inspiring, but also clearly dangerous. This, sadly, he had learned the hard way.

Midway through his second winter on Bryant road, and when still largely ignorant of his neighbour's track record, Doug Jordan approached him with a prime business prospect. It seemed while adding more insulation to his kitchen walls that morning the veteran entrepreneur happened upon a short story. The newsprint was too crumpled and yellowed to read, but a picture embedded in the middle of the text was still clear: a smiling family relishing a horse and sleigh ride on a starry winter night. Immediately, as was apparently often the case with creative genius, Doug hatched a plan: he would offer this same winter joy to his fellow Muskoka residents. All he needed was a sleigh, which he had enough scraps lying around to build himself, and a horse and harness. That was where Hal came in. If willing to bankroll this part of the operation, and if not making the many other interested parties wait too long for a decision, Doug would, as a favour, "let him in on the ground floor."

When asked today about this particular undertaking Hal only shakes his head in disbelief, but as it went, he took Doug's bait. The horse and harness were acquired at his expense, Doug built a decent sleigh, Ronnie rustled up some old bails of hay, and all put the word out in Muskoka towns.

The whole thing damned near worked. Families indeed found great joy in winter sleigh rides, and for his part Doug soon became a master at 'givin'em what they wanted'. Using that newspaper picture as his guide, every night he dressed up in an old English coat complete with matching cap and scarf. On the sleigh he offered an assortment of colourful blankets, along with such merry delights as hot cocoa and hot apple cider. The capper, however, was encouraging families to sing carols, even initiating the songs with his loud, raspy voice. Toss in a few deep and perfectly-timed ho-ho-hos from the driver and riders blissfully thought they'd stepped into their favourite fairy tale.

But, as Hal would learn was inevitable, it all too soon felt apart. Somewhere in the evolution of this grand enterprise Doug and his trusty right-hand man Ronnie discovered that serving different beverages and singing with a different clientele was decidedly more profitable. More profitable, that is, until they joyfully sang their way down a steep, wooded hill one fine March evening. The long and short of it: the sleigh was a complete wreck, Hal's horse and harness vanished into the hills never to be seen again, and Doug would thereafter have had to pay any party to ride with him.

So it was Harold Scott's scepticism toward Doug Jordan took root. Several more fiascos in the years following — and Hal's generous side allowed more — strengthened this doubt beyond recovery. Truly, to this day whenever Hal sees a certain someone approaching his place in 'business-venture mode', which somehow he can always sense, the hair on the back of his neck rises. Clearly people like that had to be avoided.

For his part Doug grew quite aware of Hal's lack of enthusiasm concerning his schemes, and this was what made the issue of his winter 'guests' such a touchy one. Doug felt a duty to rid his dear neighbour of these pests, but knew he would have to be shrewd. If realizing his plan Hal would, fearing yet another disaster, order him to abandon any rescue. In the process the dear man would seal his fate to be exploited the duration of the winter, and Doug simply couldn't allow that. Poor Hal had suffered enough. Besides, what harm could possibly come in seeing two mooches on their way?

With such in mind, the very morning after Ronnie revealed Hal's plight Doug strode briskly to his neighbour's house and banged hard on the door. Seconds later a sandy-haired, fifty-something Holly Myers appeared, smiling nervously. She was wearing a green night gown and flip-flops, and as Ronnie noted, already sported at least three different colours of makeup.

"Hal around?" Doug asked gruffly.

"'Fraid not," came a high, soft voice. "He's in town with Frank doin' stuff."

"Just bet he is!" Turning away from the door a few seconds

Doug cursed under his breath. At the same time he noticed a red toque protruding from behind a distant white pine.

Putting a hand to an ample breast, Holly said, "Oh my goodness! Is something wrong?"

"You're damn right somethin's wrong! And it's just like Hal to run off when the heat's on. Did he say when he was comin' back? Or *is* he even comin' back?"

Long, pretty eyelashes fluttered. "Of course Hal'll be back. Why wouldn't he?"

"As if you don't know," Doug answered, glaring.

Holly blushed. "I *don't* know! I know nothing about this!" She watched Doug, who now kept his eyes on the snowy verandah. Leaning out the door a little farther to regain his attention, the bottom of her gown wavering slightly in the cool morning air, she said, sweetly, "Hal probably won't be much longer, though, and I've just made fresh coffee. Care for some?"

Doug slowly looked up, studied this offer a moment, then grumbled, "Suppose ... that wouldn't hurt," and with a final glance toward the pine, stepped inside.

At Holly's coaxing he took a familiar seat at the kitchen table. "I'm Holly, by the way," she said cheerfully, "Frank and I are stayin' with Hal the rest of the winter."

Doug watched her slip to the counter. "That so?"

"Frank used to work for Hal sometimes. He's a contractor." Holly came to the table with the coffee pot and, leaning over, filled two cups, slowly and smoothly. She then sat in the chair next to Doug and crossed a pair of very graceful legs. "You been friends with Hal a long time too?"

Doug shook his large frame a little, much as a lake-dunked Saint Bernard might, then spoke again in a gruff voice. "Been friends a hell of a long time. Afraid things have taken a turn for the worse of late, though. A bad turn. That's what I'm here about. Hal's seriously in the bad books of some fellas on the road, includin' myself, for money he owes us. Liable to be trouble before long." Doug eyed Holly. "I only hope you and your husband can stay safe through it all. Be a shame if either of you ... happened to be in the wrong place at the wrong time."

Holly again blushed. "My goodness! You mean we could get hurt? Things are really that bad?"

"And not likely to get better the rest of the winter. Times are damn tough right now, and somebody not payin' him can really put a guy on edge. To hear the thoughts goin' through the heads of these boys right now ... I gotta tell you, it scared me." Doug cast an evil stare, but it was then, probably by accident when Holly squirmed in her chair, that her gown crept up her legs slightly.

"Well, we certainly wouldn't want to get mixed up in anything. Frank says we've got enough trouble as it is."

"Best you stay clear then. Best you don't say nothin' to Hal, either."

"I won't! You look so strong. So dangerous. But oh! Maybe that's the wrong thing to say. I'm so sorry."

"No, you could say ... I'm sort of ... dangerous," said Doug, and involuntarily he found his chest expanding slightly.

"Frank's not nearly so strong," Holly continued, studying her guest's large forearm. "And to think you're right next door ..." She lifted her bright blue eyes to Doug's, and he responded by shakily sipping his coffee.

During the remainder of his visit, which somehow stretched another hour, Doug shared with Holly a number of stories of past incidents of Bryant road trouble. Like the time some of the boys, who Doug dared not name, burnt a fellow's house down for welching on a poker debt. Or the night Doug himself, single-handedly, had to stop three men from emptying a woman's house of furniture as a debt payment. He also made sure to end each tale with, "But you wouldn't think anything like that would happen again, would you?"

For her part Holly kept Doug's coffee cup full, continuing to pour it ever so slowly and smoothly, and expressed her shock at regular intervals. So animated at times was this shock that often Doug lost his place in a story and retold parts. At last, however — despite Holly's expressed eagerness to hear more violent stories — he rose to leave. "Come back anytime," his host sweetly offered as he stepped out, once again hanging out the door, and by this time Doug had no choice but to turn and watch her wave goodbye.

Doug no sooner got his boots off than Ronnie was pounding on his back door, then letting himself in.

Wild-eyed, he said, "So? Scare her pretty good, Doug? Is she packin' it up already?"

Doug stared at him dazedly a moment, then proudly declared, "She's pretty much there, Ronnie. All but in tears at the end."

"Ha!" Ronnie spouted as he flaked out on Doug's homemade couch. "Figured you'd get her! Was that why she was wavin' to you as you left, Doug? Was she pleadin' for mercy —"

Doug politely broke in. "But you know — just for safe measure — we might work on the other half a bit too. What was his name again?"

"Frank."

"Sure — Frankie. We'll do a number on him too."

Ronnie suddenly sat up. "You need my help this time?"

Doug gazed out his front window, watching Hal's rusty Dodge pickup pull into its driveway, just as he had watched it pull out earlier that morning. "Not quite sure yet, Ronnie," he at last muttered harshly, deep in thought. "But be on hand. I can feel something coming."

That something took Doug about a week to develop. A trip out of town, a few phone calls, and a trap was laid. It ran basically like this: a contractor would call Frank and truthfully tell him he was looking for help in Baysville. He wouldn't specify for how long, though, and that was where Doug would step in. He would lead Frank to believe the job was a cherry and would likely last the rest of the winter. Seeing they had no transportation of their own, this would mean he and Holly would have to move to Baysville. And by the time Frank realized the job was only a two-weeker, another fellow from Bryant road would insist Hal's basement had been offered to him. It was all so basic and convenient and utterly evil that Doug kicked himself for not thinking of it sooner.

As Doug figured would happen, when Frank got the call from T. Malvis & Sons he wanted to make a trip to Baysville to scout the situation out. "Can't go jumpin' into things, Dougie my boy," he smoothly explained. Doug had this potentiality covered, however; he would drive Frankie to Baysville that very day himself. Heck, that's what neighbours were for.

But then Ronnie entered the picture.

Appearing as usual out of nowhere, he said to Doug, "Why don't I take him? I'm not doin' nothin' today."

"You don't have a truck," came a quick answer.

"We could take your snowmobile. I know the way to Baysville." Ronnie's chin rose slightly. "Been all the way to Baysville lots of times."

Doug stared into Ronnie's pleading eyes, then glanced at Frank, who now wore an even slicker grin. As sometimes happened in critical situations, he was trapped. Over the years he had seen first hand some tasks were beyond Ronnie's talents, and dealing with this Frank character seemed to fit that category. But at other times Ronnie had certainly proved very handy, and he couldn't afford losing such loyalty. So, in the end on this morning, all he could do was nod, and start worrying.

They left at noon. Ronnie drove, bundled up in all the winter clothes he could find, while Frank sat behind him, much less dressed but seemingly comfortable. Ronnie made no inquiries, occasionally catching the flash of a bottle behind him. Only ever a flash, too.

Ronnie was not outright lying to Doug when he claimed he knew the snowmobile trails leading to Baysville. He simply needed time to remember them. So despite a few wrong turns the two made decent time, following the well-groomed trails through both open fields and thick woods. The day was fresh and crisp, the sun was shining, and all seemed well. Ronnie's heart pounded at the prospect of filling such an important order for Doug.

After they had gone perhaps seven miles, however, the driver's optimism took a turn. Frank suddenly tapped him on the shoulder and asked to stop. Ronnie did so, but immediately began fretting. Breaks, he knew, begged for trouble; minds sometimes changed during breaks.

"Don't worry, Ronnie my boy," Frank perceptively offered as he lit a cigarette. I'm not having second thoughts; just thought we'd take a break. We were due for a pee and a ciggy."

To this Ronnie said nothing, only remaining seated on the snowmobile, fidgeting. It was at this time, however, Frank finally shared some of his beverage, and that made him feel a touch better. One lingering worry was the snowmobile: Frank insisted he shut it off, and now he feared it might not start again.

Doug's snowmobile had seen better days, and this was due in large part to events of several winters previous. That winter Doug started aggressively courting summer residents by phone for the job of clearing their cottage roofs of snow. He did this by substantially undercutting his competition, and such became possible through what he considered a major development in the history of roof shovelling.

In a sight several onlookers would speak of for years to come, Doug Jordan tried plowing the larger roofs that winter with his snowmobile.

Welding a small blade to the front proved no problem, and neither did getting the sled onto the roof — a cleated, wooden ramp solved that. The whole operation was, as Doug claimed to Ronnie, beautiful in its simplicity, as all great ideas were. Problem was, Doug was a big man, all of two hundred and fifty pounds, and when you added another five hundred pounds of snowmobile and who knows how much in snow load it was, as usual, simply a matter of time. As Doug later told the story, one second he was plowing a roof and the next he was sitting in the cottage's living room wiping blood from his nose. So ended that venture.

But to Ronnie's great relief, the historied snowmobile did start again, and now, after fifteen minutes of downtime, he was more than anxious to go.

Frank, however, seemed not so anxious to get on.

After curiously inspecting the bars welded to the front of the snow machine, he squinted at Ronnie through cigarette smoke. "You know, Ronnie," he began, "it doesn't seem fair."

"What doesn't —?"

"You taking most of the cold sitting up front here. Christ, what's in this trip for you?" Frank focused a piercing eye. "What say ... I drive the rest of the way?"

Ronnie pretended not to hear, using the rye as an excuse, which by this time was almost gone. When Frank only continued to stare, however, he at last said, firmly, "No way. Doug don't like nobody but me'n him drivin' his sled."

"Oh, I'm sure Doug wouldn't mind," Frank said soothingly as he handed over the last of the rye. "Besides, Doug ol' boy's not here, and the machine's pretty much done anyway, ain't it?"

"Nothin' wrong with it."

With his standard grin Frank playfully scoffed, then gently but very surely nudged Ronnie to the back of the seat. Once on himself he said, "Relax, Ronnie ol' boy. Haven't driven one of these in years, but I'm sure I'll get the hang of it."

For the first ten minutes they continued along the trail at much the same pace as before, and Ronnie started to relax. But then Frank seemed to indeed get the hang of driving again, and increased their speed. In fact, you would swear he actually started enjoying this tough chore. Becoming crazy-eyed he pushed the snowmobile to its limit, which was still plenty fast enough on a winding bush trail. On at least six occasions they very nearly crashed. "Wooo-eeeee!" Frank shouted every minute or so, and kept shouting as such for an hour before he realized Ronnie had fallen off the back.

The exact events of the rest of that afternoon Doug Jordan would never learn. All he managed to get out of Frank was that he never made it to his job interview; somehow, between all the "cruisin'" and ultimately smashing Doug's snowmobile against a tree, the gem of a job got lost in the shuffle. He was in good spirits, though, and before heading into Hal's place for a late supper, greatly relieved Doug by informing him he had not been hurt in the mishap.

As for Ronnie, it took nearly two hours of sitting in front of his woodstove before he regained feeling in his feet after his twelve-mile walk home. Doug went in to add wood and check on him numerous times over the course of the evening. On the third such visit he even found his right-hand man rocking back and forth, mumbling almost incoherently about "inecus'ble failure."

Doug did his best at comforting. "Hang in there, Ronnie," he said, his upper lip quivering. "We'll nail the bastards."

The phone call came like a dream, Doug Jordan explained to Sarah Reid back in late November of '85. A maple syrup producer in Brackenrig wanted stands to sell with his bottles of syrup that coming spring, and knew exactly where to find some. Doug's 'Pet Pine Cone' scheme several summers earlier had not realized its full potential, and he was left with some three hundred tiny 'cone beds' made of barn board scraps. Since the bottles of syrup in question weren't much bigger than pine cones, the stands would be just about perfect. Only problem was, according to the maple syrup fellow they were a touch plain. They needed sprucing up, and that, as Doug always put it, was where his new employee came in.

"Thought maybe you could paint some maple leaves on them here and there," Doug proposed one afternoon. "Between the barn boards and the leaves the bottles would look right out of the blessed sugar shack."

The whole idea seemed sensible enough to Sarah. And being out of work now several months, and with the winter only beginning, she was more than happy for any extra income. The project also suited her; in high school she had done some painting, even had a few of her works hanging in her living room that folks on Bryant road often made a fuss about.

So they began, Doug delivering the stands to Sarah's place the very day he made his offer. The A-frame she and her three kids lived in, some two miles closer to town from Doug's, was tiny but afforded enough room in back for the young woman to work. Doug stacked the stands inside the firewood porch behind the house, and Sarah would bring them in a dozen at a time to warm up before painting her maple leaves.

Doug knew a little about the young woman's situation. He didn't ask her much but he didn't need to; you could hardly sneeze on Bryant road without its residents filing a report. All knew Sarah's husband, Carl Reid, had abandoned her and the kids. He had coaxed her to Muskoka three years earlier, enticed himself by the pot of gold the area seemed, only to discover, as too many did, that certain catch to paradise. Deeply frustrated and half around the bend, he had jumped ship, leaving his wife and three young daughters to fend for themselves.

They didn't fend too well, as things went, and the family's days in Muskoka were now numbered. Sarah had already made arrangements to move back to Burlington in the spring, when a steady, year-round job would become available, but that still left the winter. With her meagre welfare income and her savings almost depleted she feared a particularly nasty season ahead, especially for her kids.

She worked long hours on the stands, as Doug knew she would. She also took great pride in them, something she was known for taking in everything she had or did, and the finished products were excellent. Indeed many leaves she made in late summer transition, skilfully having her greens give way to bright yellows, oranges, and reds. "Perfecto!" Doug told her one day, admiring one of the stands. "The buyer'll eat these up."

She painted the last of the stands about a week before Christmas, and Doug, true to his word, promptly paid her. As already arranged, Hal and Ronnie would deliver the stands to Brackenrig in Hal's truck, so they followed Doug to the Reid house the very evening Sarah said they were ready. A half hour later, with the help of Sarah's three girls, the eldest of which was twelve, Hal's capped pickup was full.

Doug then declared he needed to run some errands in town.

"If you're heading in, could I trouble you for a ride?" Sarah immediately asked. In a whisper, glancing toward the snow-covered lawn where her kids now played, she added with a smile, "I'd like to do some Christmas shopping."

"No problem at all," Doug assured her, then also offered to

bring her back in a few hours after running his errands.

When they had gone Hal backed the truck out of the driveway and, watching that he wasn't seen by Sarah's girls, who had been sent inside, he shifted into forward and started along the road, toward his place.

Ronnie turned to him. "Forget somethin' at home, Hal?"

"Yeah, a few things."

"Like what?"

"Like ... my hat."

"Your hat? Your hat's right here in the cab, Hal. Look, I've got it —"

"Nobody's waiting for us in Brackenrig, Ronnie," Hal said with a sigh, scratching his head, and didn't bother answering any more questions the rest of the way home.

It was only a matter of time, of course, before Doug Jordan hatched a new plan. He had, after all, a reputation to maintain. What might the distinguished residents of Bryant road say of him if he was outdone by a couple of good-for-nothing bums? He couldn't have it.

The solution was all so simple, it finally occurred to him: they'd merely throw a party at Hal's place, booze the two unwanteds under the table, then quietly ship them out of town. "Drink'em, Drive'em, and Dump'em," was how he eloquently described his master scheme, to which his prime helper could only gasp in awe. "Yes, I realize, Ronnie," Doug said, beaming. "It's a gift."

Hal received word he would be hosting a party only several days in advance, and naturally well after half the road knew. "High time we treated your newcomers to a proper welcome!" Doug said to him. To this Hal, knowing with word already out the party was a done deal, could only silently offer an approving nod. Also, although naturally suspecting this bash might be more than a mere welcome, what more he couldn't surmise, and he did believe in innocent until proven guilty. Nonetheless, all of this considered, he still felt certain hair rising.

The big night was the first Saturday in February. As duly

instructed the guests, all Bryant road residents, began arriving about seven. As usual with such occasions anyone and everyone showed up. But Doug did make sure a certain core group attended, even shuttling a few of these himself. Each had a reputation for being particularly enthusiastic about parties, and for having all-night stamina. "Frankie might out-drink a couple, but not 'em all," Ronnie slyly assured Ronnie, and so they were set.

By nine Hal's small house was packed to the point where several guests stood in his bathtub for lack of any other place to stand. Not that its owner noticed; he was too busy squeezing his way through the crowd, worriedly watching over his slowly-disintegrating house. "She's still under control," the true host tried to reassure him, and so while Ronnie kept the music going Doug met Frank and Holly's every need, including keeping their glasses full.

The first fight broke out about eleven. Two Bryant road boys were in dispute of late over a plowing contract, and as the beers went down things escalated. One, in fact, at last decided to plow the other right through the living room wall, and this favour was returned by a free trip through Hal's TV set. For several minutes chaos ensued, with Ronnie holding back a frantic Hal while Doug jumped into the fray to break things up. Being such a big man he was not long in doing that, and soon had a hushed combatant firmly under each hefty arm and was smiling through a cut lip at Frank and Holly. "Think nothin' of her, folks. Just having a little fun, these two." But any worries he had the celebrities of the evening might be put off by this incident were soon assuaged. While a now half-in-the-bag Holly applied bandages to the various parties, Frank cracked open another bottle of rye. Doug was pleased.

The night wore on, with yet more party-goers arriving. Soon as many stood on Hal's snow-packed lawn as in the house. Frank and Holly lapped it up, and drank steadily. They'd no sooner finish a drink than Doug or Ronnie would graciously hand them another. Problem was, they had no trouble saying thank you. Indeed, when the clock struck two Frank could have still carried on a fairly intelligent conversation, if he could have found someone. "May need to 'nitiate the backup procedure, Ronnie," Doug told the deejay, who by this time was working by feel only.

The 'backup procedure' was to get Frank into a drinking game, and what better, Doug earlier considered, than darts. For all the dust Ronnie might have had in his attic, he was awesome at darts, even plastered; 'Frankie' wouldn't know what hit him.

But he actually proved quite a capable dart player. Turned out he had played in a pretty solid Toronto league a few years, and when Ronnie finally slumped to the floor he took to showing his skills from halfway across the living room. Before several guests tackled him he even managed to score bull's-eyes on three watercolour ducks gracing Hal's dining room wall.

In the end, Doug's entire master plan unravelled. Once semi-recovered, Ronnie seemed to adopt an 'if you can't beat'em, join'em' attitude and wound up on the roof with Frank, taking turns blowing an old trumpet they'd dug out of Hal's closet. This was followed by roof-jumping, a Bryant road standard, and by streaking. About this time, too, several pickups began racing on the road, and one wound up crashing into Doug's truck, the intended 'Dump'em' vehicle. Not that the owner noticed. Only twenty minutes later a news-carrying Frank discovered him in the hall closet with Holly, wedged in the narrow space between the wall and the water heater. And although the husband's first reaction might have been high regard for their creativity, his second was, quite simply, to end Doug's life. The fight that ensued was even more vicious than the first, the two men trading blows while Holly smacked both with one of her shoes. Who knows, too, how long they might have continued if not for the approaching sirens ...

Hal Scott woke in early afternoon to water dripping through his broken roof onto his forehead. He rose, sore in more places than he could count, and with no memory of how he ended up in his bed. Perhaps he had gone there in his stupor, and perhaps he had been carried. No matter.

He limped into what was left of his living room. Ronnie was flaked out in the armchair, his face and arms still covered in soot from battling the fire. That had started when several party-goers decided to build a bonfire on the lawn; only an hour later Hal's shed lit on fire from drifting sparks. Sprawled on the floor in front of Ronnie were Vick Nelson and Jerry Howard, the abstaining driver and backup driver for Doug's scheme. Ultimately they'd abstained until about midnight, when the temptation became too great. It had been them bombing up and down the road, and only by what Doug described as a "holy Bryant miracle" had they eluded the police. As for that mastermind himself, he lay snoring on the ripped couch, a beer bottle still clutched in his hand. When Hal went by him his neighbour politely passed wind and rolled over.

The house was chilly, and he soon discovered why. One of his small kitchen windows was broken; through it protruded the tip of a snowmobile ski. But when Mr. Jordan woke he would have that "fixed in a flash," of course, so Hal merely left it.

Frank and Holly were nowhere to be seen, but Hal soon noticed a note on the kitchen table. "Thanx so much. Be in touch," was all it said. He carefully folded the scrap of paper and slipped it into his half-torn shirt pocket. Later, as a reminder, he'd transfer it to an envelope hidden in his dresser, one slowly accumulating cash to repay a loan from his bankruptcy days, but saved when his lenders accepted room and board instead. He supposed he would have to send some of that money now.

Taking a seat at the table he stared at the snowmobile ski, shivering. He considered making tea, decided he instead should savour the last of it, then rose to fill the kettle. Standing at the sink he saw a robin suddenly land on an old washer a certain neighbour had coaxed him into buying. Seeing the bird, a perennial sign of spring, he took a deep breath, and thanked God.

5

YEARS AND YEARNINGS

Young Alex Bennett could scarcely believe his eyes when he first saw the boulder. Kneeling near the lake's edge he watched, entranced, as the shadowy figures, the seemingly endless, drifting, flashing shapes played across the rock's smooth face. But although so amazed, he did not wake his grandfather napping nearby; "pure silliness" he would surely hear. He would, as always, leave the aged man to his dreamings, to the precious wonders of his past.

The summer of 1992 began badly for Alex. Bussed off against his will in early July by his mother, he was to spend the summer in Muskoka with his paternal grandparents. It was all their idea, his mother contended; "high time the boy lived a spell with his true elders" his grandfather reportedly argued by phone. And so the eleven-year-old had gone. Two months among old folk living in old houses surrounded by old trees. He knew it was cruel and disrespectful to think of his grandparents and their ever-present neighbour this way, but he saw little value in this particular experience. A short visit, as with past seasons, was one thing, but an entire summer was sure to be torture.

Jack and Hatty Bennett's home was a rocky two acres near

Milford Bay, a tiny village on Lake Muskoka. Their house was a white two-storey nestled among large pines and was built on the "aged bones of Mother Earth," meaning that rugged Precambrian foundation serving all Muskoka. Behind the house was a large workshed in which Jack once earned a living as a cabinetmaker, and in which the aged bones of ninety-one-year-old Noel Manson now resided, his apartment converted out of half this building.

Together these elderly adults would serve as Alex's only companions for the summer. No kids of similar age lived nearby, and his Native Indian grandmother would never consider allowing her one and only grandchild to stray far. "If we lose you then who will we pass our stories on to?" Hatty often asked him, always smiling and seemingly kidding. But truly she was not. Listening to stories would easily earn title to her grandson's most common pastime this summer.

One tradition established early after Alex's arrival in late June — the very day of his arrival, in fact — was afternoon fishing. This was Jack Bennett's doing; he had a favourite spot on the shore of Lake Muskoka to fish, a tiny, grassy clearing where the shoreline bedrock formed a natural bench. Here he would draw his grandson each day for several hours of casting. They rarely caught many fish, mind you, but why they always returned was soon no mystery to Alex. Each outing his dear grandfather seized the opportunity to tell stories of "the old days." Specifically, his tales were of pioneering times, and inherited from early family who in the late 1860's braved a move from Philadelphia to Huntsville. Jack had received and titled countless such stories, and during this summer Alex heard many more than once. On at least three outings, for instance, he was treated to 'The Brutal But Blessed Logging Days'. Despite this he never complained; his sentence had been handed down and he would 'serve it like a man'. His grandfather at least told his stories modestly. Indeed, he invariably closed a tale with, "But I'm not braggin' here. I'm just *sharin'*." So the boy would simply fish, and listen.

The day Alex discovered the boulder was one in early July. That afternoon he and his grandfather made their usual journey to the lake shortly after lunch. The walk took a full twenty minutes, but this time spoke more of Jack Bennett's aged, limping gait than of the distance from the Bennetts' house, which sat only a quarter-mile away.

On this bright and hot afternoon Alex ultimately went for a swim. His grandfather, as often he did, fell asleep after his fishing and story-telling (on this day the feature tale was 'The Tedious Chore of Wall Chinking') and becoming typically bored with catching few fish, Alex took to the water. Having noticed the boy was a strong swimmer Jack never minded him doing this without direct supervision, and naturally the old man would wake if any trouble arose. Alex had also learned the hard way that if he were to wake his grandfather it had better be genuine trouble; prosaic and practical right to his own rugged foundation, Jack Bennett was not one for nonsense.

And so it was this day, when Alex made his astonishing find, he didn't bother waking his grandfather. Even directly confronted with the discovery the old man would never have believed it.

Swimming farther from the "fishing bench" than he normally dared, Alex slowly crept ashore, stepping carefully on the smooth, wet bedrock. A mink was what drew his attention, but by the time he was on shore the tiny animal had long disappeared. While returning to the water and trailing his hands over several rocks, however, something else caught his attention.

The shoreline boulder was not large as boulders go, perhaps three feet wide by two high, and otherwise indistinguishable from thousands of others strewn along the shores of Muskoka lakes. In light of such normalcy, Alex first supposed what he saw to be mere shadows, a product of overhead tree branches swaying in the afternoon's light breeze. But not only did there prove to be few overhead branches at this spot, the breeze on this day was not steady, and the figures and patterns continued changing even when the air was still.

Completely bewildered, Alex could only kneel and watch.

The images followed a sequence, he soon surmised, and seemingly it began with small, dark ovals moving rapidly, and in different directions, across the boulder's broad face. These gave way to much slower ovals, some of the same size as those appearing first and some larger. Three dark, oblong figures next became visible, two large and one small, and remained motionless. What followed Alex found even less discernible; tall, shadowy spikes, dome-like figures, and tiny points of bright light drifting upward. During these particularly puzzling images Alex couldn't resist touching the boulder, placing a trembling hand against its face. To his further amazement, his hand had no effect; the images continued undaunted.

Then, all at once, they ceased; the face of the stone returned to its normal silvery-gray, and remained so as Alex continued looking on, by now utterly dazed. When at last he regained his senses he became conscious again of the lake sloshing against the shore, and just over it the distant call of his grandfather.

In what would have been a second guest bedroom on the upper floor of the Bennetts' house was a small library. The books, faded and tattered and seemingly as old as their owners, were highly treasured by Jack, Hatty, and Noel. It was their cherished collection of "books of Muskoka's olden times," times both within their lives and beyond. Alex learned early the halo surrounding these volumes; leaving one out of place — or, God forbid, actually removing one from the room — could earn cold stares all supper long. Nonetheless, for sheer lack of anything else to do he often perused the library, particularly during mornings his grandparents went grocery shopping in Bracebridge and he was confined to the house.

Many of the books were about Muskoka's grand hotels, resorts that flourished before the age of the automobile and when steamships plied the district's larger lakes. These were Noel Manson's. Both he and his parents had spent many years working at various hotels, and to this very elderly man his books were much like family photo albums.

Predictably, Jack and Hatty were not alone in sharing old stories with Alex during his Muskoka summer. Noel generally delivered his after supper, which he always had with the Bennetts, and when all retired to the front porch of the house. Having seated his ancient frame in a deck chair he would often begin spontaneously, including in the midst of others speaking, his aged ears perhaps not hearing the voices, or his mind elsewhere.

"I lived through most of what became known as the 'Golden Era' of Muskoka's grand resorts," Noel so began one evening in mid-July. "Business was still strong for the hotels when both the century and I were in our teens, and I remember well that era. With travelling much tougher folks didn't come and go so often and quickly as they do now, but usually stayed weeks on end and commonly the entire summer. Of course, generally only the wealthy could vacation for such lengthy periods; they were the hotel's main clientele, and money certainly made its mark on the times.

"Lord, what a sight these hotels were! First class in every respect. Not only were they large and ornate — with their towers and turrets and intricate trim work — but offered every manner of service and recreation you could imagine. There were ballrooms and parlours and fancy dining rooms; there were concert halls, long balconies, and gazebos by the lake. Families or young couples could golf, bowl, play tennis or croquet; they could swim, canoe, or cruise the lake in a steam yacht; they could hike trails through the woods or hire a carriage to tour the countryside. Evenings only brought more: lavish dinners and dancing and sunset strolls through the gardens.

"I remember it as truly a magical time for Muskoka; a time of grandeur, of romance. But note I *remember* it that way; back then, putting in long days as a bellhop, I found it a rather demanding time. So too my father. By the summer of '16 he was a tired man; he'd been working the hotels almost twenty years at that point. He was a gardener and took great pride in his work, but he was simply running out of steam. The gardens of the big hotels, like almost everything concerning them, required a huge effort, and such was taking its toll on his sixty-year-old frame. So much so, that after the

'16 season he intended to leave his hotel for good to pursue lighter work elsewhere.

"As chance would have it, that was the season we met a young Kingston businessman named Joseph Kensington. It was his first stay at our hotel but we already knew a few things about him. We knew, for instance, this was his third year visiting Muskoka with his sister, and also that in his two previous seasons, even only staying several weeks, he had developed something of a reputation. It seems he'd been exceptionally enthusiastic about all facilities and activities offered by his two former hotels. He was invariably the first guest up in the morning and the last to bed. Most notable, though, was how he greeted new guests. A steamer whistling in was always a festive occasion, with often half a hotel's staff and guests crowding the dock to meet those arriving. Joseph, though, was especially welcoming, shaking hands and speaking with virtually everyone. So my father and I heard, even after a steamer left this man sometimes remained on the dock, smiling broadly and searchingly, as though in utter disbelief more would not be visiting.

"When Joseph arrived at our hotel in June of '16, yet again with his sister, the two were set to spend the entire season. With his reputation preceding him this obviously came as no surprise to any of the staff. A spry and seemingly always smiling man, his energy for engaging in hotel recreations continued, and so too his dock greetings. My father and I were greatly surprised, therefore, when after only two weeks at the hotel Joseph and his sister announced they were cutting short their stay. On merely their third Saturday, in fact, they would leave the hotel.

"We were not long in learning why, nor in learning this was the third season the two had 'cut short' an intended full-summer stay. It seemed Joseph's sister, Melissa, felt it necessary to offer our hotel management an explanation for the pair's early departure, and, as spicy information was apt to do, it eventually spread through the rest of the staff. Although neither of us were much for gossip, it was inevitable my father and I would also learn of Joseph's plight. Indeed only two days passed before we overheard some chambermaids chatting during their break.

" 'And here all this time, all these summers, he's been expecting her to join him, but she's never arrived. That's so sad,' one said, to which an elder maid grumbled, 'Yes, and for the life of me I don't understand the woman's concern.'

" 'The woman', we soon learned, was Joseph's wife. Apparently each summer she had refused to join him in Muskoka because she feared it too backwoods. But each season she also hinted she might change her mind — a cousin could escort her if she did — and so Joseph had always gone ahead to Muskoka. However, with now a third occasion of his wife failing to arrive as expected — and this time at arguably the finest hotel the region had to offer — it seemed he was forced to resign.

"On his last evening my father and I wound up speaking to him. I often helped Dad water the gardens during evenings, and we were in the midst of catering to some lilac bushes when Joseph approached us.

" 'I'm leaving tomorrow for Kingston,' he said brightly, holding out a hand to both of us, 'and I wanted to thank you two. Melissa and I have had a wonderful stay.'

"Both Dad and I politely told him he was welcome, and then watched him gaze lovingly at the hotel. 'I intended to bring my wife to Muskoka,' he said as he did so. 'I'm certain she would have enjoyed it here.'

"My father said, warmly, 'Perhaps another year she'll come.'

" 'Yes, perhaps she will,' Joseph echoed, and his gaze now turned to the hotel's dock, where here and at others he had so many times waited for that wife to come.

"At last he again turned to my father and me, and, his eyes vacant and his smile somewhat pained now, said, 'I was hoping to spend the entire summer here. I love Muskoka very much.'

" 'Yes,' Dad said, studying Joseph closely, 'it is a pleasant place.'

"He spoke with Joseph about another ten minutes that evening before the Kingston man continued his walk, before he thanked yet more staff members, before he indulged in a final swim. Much of his conversation with my father was light and common — they spoke of the hotel's boats, of the fine Muskoka lamb served in the

dining hall that evening, of the vines covering the railings of the
verandahs, of lake views at sunrise. Yet there was something about
Joseph making their conversation special. Whenever he spoke of
the hotel there was an unmistakable sparkle in his eyes, one unlike
I'd seen in any other guest. Even at the age of fifteen I sensed how
deep his feelings were for Muskoka, and his gaze I would never
forget. Perhaps that look is even most responsible for my saying
tonight the grand hotel era was magical. Apparently, too, I was not
the only one struck by Joseph Kensington's sparkling eyes.

"As planned, he left with his sister on the steamer the morning
following our talk with him. My father and I saw him off, then
never saw them again. Others did come the following year, though,
and I heard many comment the gardens looked especially lovely
that season."

At every opportunity Alex visited the boulder. With his
grandfather's fishing naps often short, however, such opportunities
were rare. But he did manage a fairly lengthy visit in late July, and
what he discovered only added to the boulder's mystery.

The afternoon was overcast and dim, and when Alex reached
the boulder he was not long in noticing something new. After
gently touching it, which by now he had learned was necessary, not
only did the boulder display figures and patterns, but also it
occasionally changed colours. At once it was gray, then blue, then
red; ultimately it seemed to pass through almost the entire
spectrum. As when first discovering the boulder Alex considered
himself possibly mistaken, but after several minutes of close study
he found he was not: the boulder was truly changing colours. Again
he could only sit, completely entranced, watching until hearing his
grandfather's call.

In the midst of such visits to the boulder, Alex naturally
continued listening to his grandfather's stories of Muskoka's
pioneering times, the era preceding that of the grand hotels. He

would usually lie back in the soft grass behind the stony bench during such tales, paying little mind to his fishing. Doing so seemed to please his grandfather, the elder taking satisfaction in having his grandson's undivided attention. Indeed, as the summer progressed Alex increasingly noticed the pleasure assumed by all the story-tellers surrounding him. "We consider your ears a gift," Noel once declared, and the young man gradually came to understand.

So he did at the lake one fine afternoon in early August when Jack delivered a story about his pioneering great-grandmother. Alex already knew from past family stories that Jack thought fondly of Stella Bennett, and if ever he would indulge in fanciful thoughts it was concerning this matriarch. As always he gave her story a name, this one entitled, 'Of Mud and Grace'.

"Stella was not of a rugged sort, unlike how most folk seem to think all settlers were," Jack started with, all but ignoring his fishing line now. "She was frail, city-raised, and used to going to tea parties, not hoeing fields. Most who knew her were bloody amazed Jim and Irene Garvey intended to move this fourteen-year-old daughter from Philadelphia to a muddy, mosquito-infested lot in Canada. What they didn't realize, though, is the huge opportunity her parents, and especially her father, saw in Muskoka; the family would move, snatch up all kinds of free land, and live far better than they ever had in Philadelphia. They could see the makings of a dream.

"As you might guess, things sure as hell didn't work out that way; farming for the Garveys, like for most in Muskoka, proved a bust. Jim did manage to build the family a decent house — by settler standards, at least — but his money soon ran out. By their third autumn, when Stella turned seventeen, both he and Irene were forced to find other work. For Jim this meant a lumber camp, dangerous and gruelling work that would keep him away from home months at a time. Irene, meanwhile, was lucky enough to land a job as a clerk in a Huntsville general store.

"The owners of the store, Ned and Paula Dobson, were from Britain, and money-wise had done relatively well in Muskoka. Paula's health was another matter, and hired help in the form of Irene was a luxury she'd long looked forward to. Over the years of

working the store the British woman started suffering more and
more back problems, and unable to move around much she gained
a ton of weight. When Irene began work at the store Paula was
every bit as heavy as herself, and the Garvey mother was a large
woman. Just how much Paula had changed was evident by a grainy
photograph of her and Ned tacked, perhaps in boast, on the wall
behind the store's front counter. It was taken the day the couple
arrived in Canada, and showed a svelte Paula in a lovely afternoon
dress, a green garment her employee later saw and could hardly
believe how undersized it now was. Financially secure as the
Dobsons may have been, Muskoka had clearly taken its toll on them
also, and this fact restored some of Irene's pride after the Garveys'
failure in farming.

"Irene walked about seven miles to the general store each day,
leaving for Huntsville at dawn and often not returning until almost
nightfall. With Jim also away this left Stella alone at the family's
remote homestead, and clearly this was not a life she was suited to.
Finished school, unable to find work, and with no close neighbours,
she soon became extremely lonely. She loved her parents, and
respected their attempt to make a better life for the family, but often
she considered they'd be better off returning to Philadelphia, even
broke. Despite the noise and pollution, at least in the city there
were streets and buildings and neighbours nearby. But she was not
one to complain and so never said anything to Jim or Irene. She did,
however, secretly treasure one item reminiscent of her former life.

"It belonged to her mother, who kept it neatly tucked in a box
in her bedroom cabinet. Irene considered the red dress the finest
she'd ever owned, and was determined to keep it regardless of how
financially challenged the family became. She therefore kept it
hidden in her cabinet, knowing Jim never dared venture inside.

"Stella, though, knew about the dress. She and her much larger
mother had a few clothes they could share, and she happened upon
the dress one typical afternoon spent alone in the house. In time she
even tried it on, and from there formed a habit. She told my
grandmother, from whom I heard this story, that she felt silly but
couldn't help herself. The garment was far too big for her, of

course, but it was, nonetheless, an elegant, lace-trimmed dress, and entirely in contrast to the rough and raw world of pioneering Muskoka. Often she would stand in front of her mother's small bedroom mirror, posing and even imagining herself at a tea party back in Philadelphia. Or maybe at a dance, or a fancy city restaurant. The dress, simply put, became an escape for Stella, and silly or not, one dearly needed.

"The family's third Christmas in Muskoka was a modest occasion, as all knew it would be. Although working, Jim had not yet been paid, and Irene's wages were minimal. Coupled with the plight of their original savings the family's holiday proved their most meagre ever, and it showed on them. As the three sat together in the house's main room after a bare-bones Christmas supper all were quiet and somber. At last Jim, rising to fetch more firewood, said to Stella, 'I'm sorry, Dear, that ... we've now so little.' And when he was gone Irene also soon rose to busy herself with chores, but she, oddly, said nothing.

"Several days later, with Jim already back at the lumber camp, Irene rose just before dawn to ready herself for a return to work. As usual Stella prepared breakfast — on this day oatmeal and biscuits — but unlike most mornings she and her mother remained silent as they ate. There was a heaviness to the room, and Stella was undeniably relieved when her mother donned her coat and boots. Watching her slowly trod through the snow, Stella softly said from the door, in desperation, 'I thought we had a wonderful Christmas, Mother. Thank you so much.'

"At this Irene turned and offered a reply her daughter found curious. With a slight grin even, she said, 'I, for one, don't believe Christmas is quite over yet.' With that she carried on toward town.

"Stella was not long in understanding.

"That very morning, in an effort to raise her spirits, she made her way up to her parents' bedroom, intent on finding escape in the usual manner. But on this occasion, when she opened the box where Irene stored her prized red garment she found it missing. Instead, in its place was a green dress, one with P.D. embroidered inside the collar, and it fit Stella perfectly."

Alex was "old" before he received official word his paternal grandmother was part Native Indian. He had, however, long noticed differences in her appearance from most adults he knew, and by them had been fascinated — the satiny, midnight black hair; the dark complexion; the sharpness of her face and frame. He had also witnessed, even at a tender age, a rare strength of will, and dark eyes that could often seem vacant and yet miss nothing. But not until one afternoon when he was nearly eight, and immediately following a story his grandmother told to a gathering in his family's Sarnia house, did she quietly but firmly tell him of her heritage.

Her message, like everything about her, was direct: she was proud to have within her Indian blood, proud to be born of a people who had lived in this land we now call Muskoka for thousands of years, and most especially, proud to maintain and forward traditional beliefs. Others, she said, glancing toward the living room, could scoff or snicker all they wanted; she respected their beliefs, could they not do likewise?

Those words stayed with Alex. From that day forward he viewed his grandmother as one for whom all was open to possibility, one for whom there was no 'real' world but endless worlds. And yours was as valid as hers.

"He seemed to appear out of nowhere, this young man," Hatty began one morning in mid-August. Seated near her large kitchen window she watched several nuthatches weave through the aged pines behind the house. For a moment her usually dark, vacant eyes flickered, then almost glowed as she looked skyward.

"The women were sewing moccasins, the special kind of the Ojibwe, when he stumbled into the clearing. His entire lean, tanned body was dripping with sweat and his eyes were distant and crazed. They laid him down in one of the wigwams, where they gave him some water, and where after some time he spoke.

"He had been out deer hunting since dawn. Many other men joined him, but as the morning brightened they strayed farther and farther from one another. The young man also stopped to rest at one point, for he was a little tired on this day. By the time he continued through the forest he had lost sight of the others, and when he called to them he heard no answer.

"He began to wander, more concerned now for finding his fellow hunters than for hunting. The forest he was in was mostly pine, and they were the giants that lived before the time of the white man. Their tops were so thick the light was dim even in midday. He walked through this dark forest for a long while, becoming more and more worried. The others would laugh at him for getting lost, even though the group was in an area unfamiliar to them, and he did not want to be laughed at.

"His spirits rose when he reached a bright clearing with a small pond in the middle. He would build a fire here, add some wet leaves, and perhaps the others would see the smoke and come to him. He would say he intended to find a place like this, and so they would not laugh at him.

"As he gathered dry twigs, though, he saw something peculiar about the clearing. The bark on the pines surrounding it was yellowish, unlike he had ever before seen. Some plants growing at the edge of the pond he had also never before seen — tall, woody plants with spear-shaped leaves and thorny roots protruding from the ground. To see such new things he found odd, of course, for he had lived in the forest his entire life. What even more surprised him — and frightened him — was when a large beaver suddenly surfaced in the pond, and when he moved close it stayed still and did not dive. It simply watched him.

"He ran from the clearing into the dark forest again, and ran until his heart almost pounded through his chest. Being young and strong he could run a very long time, and so must have gone a very long way. At last, though, he tripped over a fallen tree branch and hit his head on the hard ground.

"He said he must have been knocked unconscious because he next remembered it feeling much later in the day. He was at the edge of another clearing, this one even larger, and he should have again been in the sun. But instead, when he rolled onto his back he saw the sky was a deep red, and from greenish clouds hung braided ropes made apparently of moose hair. He thought he was dying. He became more scared than ever before in his life, and again he ran.

"At last he reached the clearing where the women sewed, and was relieved when he saw they were normal and so too the sky and trees and a stream flowing nearby. The women also did not laugh at his story, but listened. They listened knowing many mysteries remained in the world, and seeing no reason this young man would lie. When he fully recovered he seemed normal; he was not crazy. And so they believed.

"This was their way, the Indian way."

The next several weeks of that summer passed quickly for Alex, as the final weeks of summer vacations invariably did. During this time he continued visiting the boulder whenever he could, and sensed, as peculiar as it seemed, that it too knew time was running out. There was an urgency to the shadowy figures and colours now; they flashed across the boulder's face more rapidly, and the same sequences were thus repeated more often during each of Alex's visits. It was, it seemed, as though the boulder was trying to tell him something, and knew it was not succeeding. "What are you trying to say?" he even softly whispered during one visit, not worrying, in light of his grandmother's advice, how silly such a question might have sounded. For Alex the boulder was very much real, and over the next several weeks he was consumed with finding an answer to its mysterious message.

One night during his last week Hatty Bennett entered Alex's room to check on him. She found the boy sound asleep, as she expected, but with his night table lamp still on and a large book open and facedown on his chest. Recognizing immediately it belonged to the sacred library in the adjacent room, she sighed and gently pulled the book from her grandson's limp hands. She looked at it a moment before closing and placing it on the night table. She then drew the covers up to Alex's chin and forgivingly pecked his forehead. As she left the room she also did not take the book but tucked it under a small cloth covering the table, only the spine remaining unhidden: 'A Stroll Through Time: Muskoka's Countless Faces'.

It was several evenings later, and only two days before he was to return home, that Alex made his final visit to the boulder that summer. For over an hour after his grandmother came in to check on her 'sleeping' grandson he waited for the house to quiet, then another half-hour for safe measure. Removing from his window the framed screen he had earlier studied, he slowly climbed onto the porch roof, then hung from its edge and dropped the last four feet to the ground. A mere ten minutes later, miraculously without rousing any of the dogs in the area, he succeeded in getting to the lake.

The moon was in its first quarter on this evening and offered little light, but Alex found the boulder without trouble. Kneeling, he gently touched the ancient stone. For a moment nothing happened, however, and he feared all was lost. But at last the sequences of figures and patterns began as always, although in the darkness they were much clearer against their colourful backdrops.

And Alex also knew now what each was.

The powerboats, those he had unknowingly watched many times before as dark ovals, cruised playfully across the lake on this bright, cloudless day. When their waves reached shore they lapped the base of the boulder, and also bobbed the floats of two nearby fishermen, an aged man and a young boy. The boy lay back while his elder remained upright, gazing at distant, cottage-sprinkled shores. Alex could just make out his face, his moving lips.

The slower boats again came next, and these now clearly made of wood, their deeply-finished mahogany gleaming in the sun. In them sat men and boys in yachting whites and straw hats, women and girls in lace-trimmed dresses of lawn or muslin. All were smiling and festive. Some shared waves with a uniformed chambermaid lunching next to the boulder, the young woman in turn watching the approach of a distant steamship.

A team of oxen pulling a plow followed, and a farmer stooped to dip a tin cup into the lake. He drank quickly, and often, and several times wiped his brow with a torn shirt sleeve. Behind him were mostly cleared but rocky, patchy fields, and not once did the farmer turn to look at them. He remained kneeling by the water, peering at his reflection, at his dishevelled hair and tired, worn face.

Soon, however, enormous trees rose on this same land, a thick forest of towering white pines, and near shore now stood a young boy in deer skins. He too drank from the lake, but with cupped hands, and peacefully. It was evening, a half moon glowed in the deep black of the sky, and between two wigwams a small fire burned. Around it several men, richly adorned in feathers and furs, danced while others looked on, all faces reverent and appearing in flashes amid the fire's rising sparks.

And then all at once the entire boulder turned a rich blue, and from its base tiny bubbles slowly drifted upward to the distant surface of what Alex knew was Lake Algonquin. The boulder remained this blue almost a minute while fish energetically darted over its face, fish large and healthy, and abundant.

Next came a series of colours. Four times the boulder alternated between a mottled green and brown, and an icy blue. During one such transition Alex watched an image of the boulder being cleaved into existence, along with others, a ridge of bedrock clearly yielding to the enormous force of an advancing glacier.

Eventually the boulder again turned entirely blue, but this time a lighter shade, that of the sea. The fish shadows Alex now saw were more varied in size, and often displayed shapes he had never before seen. Soon, though, the boulder began to vibrate, which Alex could feel through his feet and when he reached out to touch the boulder. Soon also, on its face, he watched fissures form in a worn and barren moutainscape.

The images and colours became stronger now, the boulder seemingly ever more energized. Its vibrations strengthened; in silhouette came images of exploding lava, and mountains rising. So intense did this display become that Alex had difficulty making sense of dozens of images. At last, though, all ceased, and out of the darkness the boulder gradually brightened to an orange-red, so bright Alex needed to shield his eyes. And he now knew what he was witnessing.

In time the boulder grew dark again, and from then on, for Alex, remained that way. But perhaps, he years later reflected, a day would come when it would again tell its own story of Muskoka, of all it had seen of this land through the depths of time. If only coming upon another with whom it could share.

6

The Journey Home

"Wasn't all it was cracked up to be, was it now?"

Stan Keswick grinned all-knowingly while uttering these words to his son, and the son felt a familiar twinge.

"No, Dad," Loren Keswick tiredly answered, gazing at the boring and beloved neighbourhood spread out below him. "I suppose it wasn't."

The two men were, as often so on clear summer nights, perched atop the Keswicks' Bracebridge townhouse. A decade earlier, on a whim his dear wife Mary thought, or hoped, a temporary fit of insanity, Stan built a platform on the backyard side of the roof, accessed from the attic by a small hatch. Using old lumber so his wife wouldn't have cost as firepower, he built the whole thing in an afternoon. "For sitting out at night. What's wrong with that?" he argued, to which Mary smartly replied, "For tripping one night and falling headfirst thirty feet to the ground, you mean." But foolhardy as it may have been, and despite stares from sidewalk passers-by, who occasionally caught sight of the platform through the maples lining the Keswicks' corner lot, Stan persisted. Indeed as the years passed he came to treasure his private little perch and would now never even consider parting with it. It was where he did his thinking, where "he sorted out his hand."

Or, such as on this night, someone else's.

"Have you looked much for another apartment yet? You hated the place you were in, but you went right back to it."

"Just got home, and maybe it's not so bad."

"Just got home, huh? Your boss and I once renovated this whole house in the same time that's passed since you got home."

Loren looked to the street, where a woman walking her dog was peering upward. "Then I guess I simply haven't found the energy or concentration to decide yet. But I will."

"You're still licking your wounds, is what you're saying." Stan smirked. "Sorry for rubbing it in so much, but you have to admit what happened is exactly what I said would happen. You've learned I was right."

Quietly, and once again wearily, Loren answered, "Yes, I learned."

It had been several months now since he returned from travelling the world, two months of digesting and regrouping, of trying to decide what went right and what went wrong, and which was which. Looking back to the true beginnings of this journey, however, he wondered, even with his father's warnings, whether things could have gone any other way. Whether, that is, it would have even been possible for him to see his quandary coming.

He was only twenty when he first left home. Fresh out of high school several friends approached him with the prospect of a European tour, a special they'd seen in the window of a travel agency. With a few thousand dollars saved from summer jobs, and no interest in college or university, he needed only several days to reach a 'why not' decision. Too, once briefed his parents had little problem with the idea, the trip, after all, being only a month long and through a reputable tour company. "It's the age for crazy, spur-of-the-moment adventures," he overheard his mother say to his father one evening. So off he went.

Predictably, the tour, comprised almost entirely of people his age, proved as much a rolling party as an exploration of Europe. Nevertheless he was smitten by the basic experience of encountering new places and new people, including those from the many countries represented in the tour group, and returned home wild-eyed and endlessly talking. Out of sympathy for the neighbours his father eventually even temporarily revoked his platform privileges.

When the dust at last settled on that first trip — when he had shown his photos to any and all willing, copied his travel journal for safekeeping, and told every story nineteen times — life, as it was bound to, returned to normal. Or so he expected.

Over the next several years he grew increasingly conscious of, and frustrated by, a routineness and tedium to his life. Working long hours as a fireplace mason, a trade handed down by his father, and forever surrounded by the same landscape and people, he found one day merely blended into the next. He was living in a blur. Reflecting on his trip to Europe, he found it both odd and depressing he could recount every single day of two weeks several years earlier but had difficulty recounting even the most recent two weeks since. So quickly, also, had those recent weeks passed. "It's the richness of your life's experience that dictates the flow of time, not the calendar" he once read, and he came to see truth in this. One evening after supper he said to his mother, "It's as though when I'm travelling I'm alive, and when I'm at home I just exist." Seeing her eyes quickly sadden he instantly regretted his comment. But in his heart he held to what he said, and merely a year later, having pulled together a decent amount of money, he announced to his parents he would do another trip. A much longer trip, one taking him around the world, and on his own.

This time his parents were not so supportive.

His father was most outspoken, and although not hindering Loren his message was clear: the young man would regret this trip. He would travel, realize the rest of the world was not quite as amazing as he thought, and end up right back where he started. Meanwhile all he had saved, enough for a down payment on a small house, would be lost. Stan also had a pretty good track record of proving right.

But Loren, like that very father, ironically, was unswayable.

He left on a rainy Wednesday in early June, his parents seeing him off at the airport in Toronto. His mother, as he feared she might, shed tears and his father was quiet and somber. For a moment Loren wondered whether he was in fact making a huge mistake. Later, in the departure lounge, he did little but stare out at the rain-soaked tarmac.

Once airborne, however, he soon got over this anxiousness, and convinced himself his hardy parents would too. After all, he was off! A full year of travelling the world. Even now, fourteen months after that day, he still remembered well the excitement he had felt, the wonder over what lay ahead. Indeed he remembered his entire trip with utmost clarity. At will, it seemed, he could go back ...

Africa. The 'dark continent' proved anything but; a giant and mostly accessible land richly diverse in landscape and culture. For four months he travelled here, flying into Nairobi from Toronto via London, hitchhiking south to the tip of the continent, then in similar style but by a different route north again to Kenya. He first heard about the hitchhiking approach from a young German traveller in a dollar-a-night lodge in Nairobi. "Absolute best way to go," the fellow insisted, recently back from three months worth. Loren had hesitated; it seemed dangerous, and particularly, selfish. Who was he, who earned as much in an hour in Canada as many on this continent did in a month, to bum a ride? But he soon learned hitchhiking was virtually a form of public transportation in Africa. At the end of a typical day he had often spent more contributing to gas during his rides than he would have on bus fares. As for the danger element, after noticing the miserable condition of the average African bus, and how it was driven, he felt he was taking serious risks either way, so on he hitched.

He averaged five rides a day, and encountered, seemingly, every manner of African possible, from field workers to trophy hunters to South African freedom-fighters. A mix of lush jungle, savannah, and low, rolling mountains made the scenery equally diverse. Added with never quite knowing where a hitched ride would take him — drivers were often full of ideas about where he should go — each day became for Loren a complete adventure unto itself. Often at night he would think back to the morning and the basic plan he had in mind, and then about how differently the day unfolded. He quickly came to love the freedom and spontaneity of this style of travelling, and was always up early each day eager for more.

His only break from hitchhiking was a safari out of Arusha, Tanzania. He joined three other travellers — a Danish couple and an Italian man — through a tour company. Over the next five days his group visited Tarangire, Lake Manyara, the Serengeti, and Africa's famed Ngorongoro Crater. During this time he saw elephant herds numbering a hundred or more, zebras, wildebeest, buffalo, giraffes, wart hogs, hippos, and seemingly dozens of species of antelope and birds. He was left mesmerized, and only wondering about the Africa that once was.

He entered Malawi, the 'Warm Heart of Africa', on a Tuesday morning in July, after just over a month of travelling. He hitched an early ride in a pickup from Myeba in Tanzania to the border, and in the back of this truck there began a series of surprises to his day. The first was meeting one of his more interesting travelling companions.

Akash, dressed in a *shalwar kameez* and sandals, was travelling from India to visit relatives in Lilongwe, Malawi's capital. He had been through a long and tough journey and was much looking forward to reaching his destination. Loren would only learn all this later, however, because the Indian could not share a single word beyond 'thank-you'. Deep within a continent whose common language was English, how this fellow had made it this far Loren couldn't fathom. But he greatly admired him for his obvious resourcefulness and determination, and so resolved to help him get to Lilongwe.

When they reached the border post Loren helped Akash fill out a form each was handed, inventing most of the Indian's background, and the two were luckily soon inside Malawi. From here, however, their forward progress came to halt, since there was little traffic. An hour passed where the two young men did nothing but quietly walk the shoulder of the road.

It was Akash who at last flagged down a large transport. When it stopped on the shoulder in a cloud of dust he ran ahead to see the driver, and before Loren in turn even reached the truck the deal, struck evidently by gestures only, was done. But as Loren approached the cab his day took another turn: Akash tugged on his arm, and pointed to the top of the truck's high, tarp-covered load.

What first seemed a terrible idea proved a tremendous one. Slowly lumbering down the highway, refreshed by the relief the breeze offered from the stifling heat, the views of Lake Malawi and its surrounding hills and plains were spectacular; seated so high they could see for miles in all directions. Occasionally they also passed through villages and, being so visible, were greeted with countless shouts and waves. Nearly four hours they travelled this way, and Loren would later consider this experience one of the highlights of his time in Africa.

In late afternoon they reached the base of the road leading up to Livingstonia, and here the two left the truck and walked to the village. It proved tiny, but after searching awhile and asking some villagers Loren found a small guest house where he and Akash could spend the night. They would not be alone: four other foreign travellers had already taken up residence for the evening. Too, one of them, an Australian named Tyler, had lived in India three years and could speak Hindi. Akash was beside himself over his incredible luck, and chatted with the Aussie for two full hours. After supper Loren received a summary.

"He told me there was trouble in his home village, and he was driven out," Tyler quietly explained. "He had no choice but to leave. It's been bloody difficult for him here, too; he speaks five languages, but not English." Tyler later added, "I've got a car and I'm going to Lilongwe tomorrow. I'll take this fellow with me. That'll free you up to do whatever you want."

So it was settled, and Loren felt happy for Akash. For his part the Indian was very grateful for his help crossing the border, which might otherwise have proven difficult, and through Tyler asked him for his home mailing address. With the aid of one of his relatives Akash would later send news of the remainder of his trip, and, Loren only supposed, another thank-you.

This, however, was when his day took a final and even more unusual turn.

Stupefied, pen and paper in hand, after several minutes worth of scratchings he could only stare at Akash and gesture with his hands his failure. Turning to Tyler he said, "Tell him ... I don't believe this. Tell him I .. simply can't remember right now."

Akash quietly spoke in Hindi to Tyler, who in turn said to Loren, "He says he's not offended if you'd rather not give him your address. He understands."

Loren's eyes bulged. "I'd be more than happy to give him my address! But I just ..."

Tyler studied him, and grinned. "Been into the local brew, Mate?"

But he obviously hadn't, and later, while joining a party with the other travellers he sensed his 'refusal' to offer Akash his address didn't sit well with them. He wound up, that is, feeling like a paranoid snob.

The party continued until about two, at least for Loren. At that time he retired to his room. It was here a thought suddenly came to him, and after removing his money belt he searched inside. Sure enough, on a small list of mailing addresses his mother had made for him she even included the Keswicks' own. In utter disbelief he stared at the familiar words and numbers a moment, then proceeded to write them on a separate piece of paper. This he would promptly give to Akash in the morning. He then switched off the light and climbed into bed. In four hours he would be up again, dressed and breakfasted by seven, and by eight at the side of the highway, thumb out ...

Asia, too, proved spectacular. About three months later, in early October, Loren found himself on this largest of continents. Flying into Karachi from Nairobi he bussed his way across Pakistan, then trekked in the Himalayas of Nepal a month before moving on to Thailand, Malaysia, Singapore, and Indonesia. His funds were holding out, with costs in most countries very low, and so too his energy, this issue the most baffling to his parents. Once a month he spoke with them by phone. "Are you not getting tired, for God's sake?" his mother always asked, and he truthfully answered he was not. Even with all he had seen and done he was still eager for more.

Visiting Irian Jaya, the Indonesian half of the massive island of New Guinea, was an idea he gained from an Argentinean traveller in the Indonesian capital of Jakarta. This largest of Indonesian provinces was reportedly among the most remote and primitive places left on Earth, with many parts of the island not fully explored. The numerous tribal peoples were barely removed from the Stone Age, with even head-hunting and cannibalism still practised in recent history. And it took Loren about five minutes to decide he had to go there.

After spending a week on the island of Lombok he flew to Biak, a tiny island off the coast of New Guinea, then took a second flight to the coastal town of Jayapura, the largest settlement in Irian Jaya. Several days later he flew into the interior, destined for the town of Wamena in the Baliem Valley.

From some reading Loren learned Irian Jaya was a curious mix of mangrove swamps, snow-capped mountains, and almost impenetrable rainforest. Many experts believed the difficulty of travel on the island, preventing native groups from having much or any contact with one another, was likely responsible for the enormous number of languages having developed here; the estimates ran from two hundred to a staggering eight hundred, almost half the languages on the planet. This difficulty in travel was also likely the reason the island's inhabitants remained cut off from the rest of the world until about the middle of the twentieth century. Up to this time natives were still using stone implements and adhering to customs and beliefs thousands of years old. Visiting Irian Jaya was very much, therefore, an opportunity to virtually step back in time.

For about an hour from his plane's window seat Loren gazed out at this peculiar land, at rugged mountains and rainforest seemingly only broken by brown tropical rivers. It was, it seemed to him, almost monotonous in this respect. But then the plane crossed a mountain peak, and at once he was over the great expanse of the Baliem Valley. The land was now mostly cleared, and below he could see clusters of wood and grass huts, and crops.

For reasons unknown to Loren the pilots left the cockpit door open, and through this doorway he watched in amazement as barely clad natives, along with livestock, scattered off the rough runway as the plane landed. "Welcome to Wamena," the Indonesian man sitting next to him said, smiling.

Loren was hardly through the formalities at the 'terminal', which seemed little more to him than a large hut itself, when he was approached by a small, lean man offering his guiding services. Having talked with the Australian in Jakarta Loren was not overly surprised at this; although tourism numbers in Irian Jaya were relatively small, the Baliem Valley was one of its 'hot spots', and he knew before coming here he would by no means be the first.

The guide's Christian name was Isaac, and Loren soon hired him. He had no choice in this respect; it was illegal to trek without a guide, and as he soon learned, probably ill-advised anyway. He also found the English of this particular guide quite good, and this was necessary for he had so far learned little Indonesian, and naturally knew nothing of the island's native languages.

The village offered only several places to stay, so deciding on a hotel was not a lengthy chore. Isaac led the way into the dusty courtyard of a small white house whose owner proved a heavy-set Indonesian man. The upstairs room he presented was basic but decent, and once settled in, Loren sat with Isaac downstairs in the main room going over plans for a trek into Lani territory, Isaac's homeland. It was here Loren soon met a stout, fifty-something American engineer named Bill Jeremy, also staying at the hotel, and also with plans of trekking. An easy-going, likeable enough man, Loren soon agreed to team up.

The following morning they visited the village's market to buy supplies for the trek. Here Loren found a surprising array of goods, including a wide assortment of vegetables — many of these in scattered piles on the ground — along with fish, clothing, shoes, and modern farming and cooking utensils. Also there were souvenir items for the growing tourist trade, such as native jewelry made of brightly-coloured feathers and boar tusks, Asmat carvings, and penis gourds, the hollow roots which served as the traditional and sole means of dress for tribal men. The people of the market, both vendors and buyers, were an equally curious mix of modern and primitive. Walking through the extremely crowded, sweaty, fly-ridden aisles Loren saw Indonesians and young natives wearing modern-style clothing — even brand-name T-shirts and shoes — alongside many older, near-naked natives. This contrast was perhaps most dramatically displayed in what Loren saw outside one of the market buildings: traditionally-dressed natives huddled around, and seemingly mesmerized by, a tiny television set.

With all supplies acquired they headed out early the following morning. The first stage of the trek was a lengthy van ride into Lani territory. Loren saw little of interest during the drive, but upon setting out on foot the marvels of this land quickly became apparent.

The first day of the trek Loren could only later remember in flashes so much did he see and experience, a day of lush, tropical mountain valleys, rain-swelled rivers, and scattered, picturesque Lani villages. Too, rivers often hosted bathers, a young boy perhaps scrubbing an elder's back, and forever upon meeting natives on the trails they were warmly greeted with the traditional "Wa!"

In late afternoon they arrived at the village where they were to spend their first night. It was comprised of five circular huts of different sizes, the walls made of slabs of wood and the roofs of thatched straw. Gathered around these huts were smiling natives of all ages, the younger, especially, taking great interest in the newcomers. Even the zippers on his rain jacket, Loren noticed, served as objects of wonder.

After spending a minute speaking to the village chief, a short, exceptionally dark-skinned man, Isaac led the way to the largest hut. Loren soon learned it, like all the others, was two-storeys, with the ceiling of the first only about four feet high. He also learned the huts had no chimneys; the smoke slowly seeped out the thatch, and the little accumulating helped repel snakes and mosquitoes.

Night soon descended, and the villagers gathered around a fire, one started, Loren noticed, by a tribesman using only sticks. Soon, as their supper of rice and noodles cooked in a large pot over this fire, Loren and Bill were treated to singing, as they would be in every village during their trek. With no apparent prompting a young boy began quietly chanting, and within seconds all had joined in, the Lani words changing with each pass of the same short melody. Several children added percussion-like sounds and the music steadily grew in complexity. Seemingly no one in the group orchestrated all this, and Loren could only watch and listen in amazement.

His sleep was broken often that first evening. Supper was served inside the hut, and drawn by odours and crumbs, many times during the night rats entered. One, in fact, even crawled over his bare chest. But also contributing to his broken sleep, unquestionably, were a thousand thoughts and experiences spinning in his head. Foremost was something from Isaac at the fire, not long before bed: "What you see is not going to last," he had somberly whispered in his ear. Loren realized he was referring to the encroaching modern world, and he also realized he was contributing to that encroachment. "The responsible traveller is forever aware he or she is not only experiencing, but *being* experienced," he had read in a travel guide, and he now painfully understood this.

For the next several weeks the group continued through the mountains, spending a few days at each village. At first all seemed quite similar, but in time Loren learned each had its own particular flavour. Indeed, some villages offered experiences he found quite peculiar.

One afternoon Loren met a woman with hardly any fingers left. From Isaac he learned that as a symbol of mourning when a relative dies, a Lani woman must have part of a finger removed. A sharp stone tool was used. An elder, this particular lady had engaged in this practice many times, and Loren wondered how she managed.

On another day, during a morning the group came upon a small market, Loren was confronted by a wild-eyed, feather-dressed man brandishing a spear. Loren froze in fear until a group of village men dragged the spear-holder away. "We are sorry — this is a madman," Isaac explained. "He has a snake in his head." Later, during lunch, surrounded by innocent but ever-staring villagers, Bill said to Loren, "It's interesting. I've talked with Isaac and learned he wasn't using an expression. He and the others wholeheartedly believe there is an actual snake in that man's head."

But most peculiar, for Loren, was an experience four days later, during their next to last evening before returning to Wamena. The village they spent this night was especially small, comprised of only three huts, but boasted a spectacular mountain view, perched as it was on a hilltop. The view was stunning enough that after removing his pack Loren spent considerable time taking it in, slowly watching the sun descend to a vast and undulating horizon.

After supper Loren and Bill crawled into their sleeping bags early, utterly exhausted. The long, hot days of mountain hiking had taken their toll, especially on the older of the two. Bill was soon fast asleep.

Loren was close to falling asleep as well when the village's chief, a shrivelled old man who looked near his time, entered the hut and took a place in front of the tiny central fire. Through a veil of smoke Loren watched as he quietly spoke with Isaac, and then as he looked sternly at his guests. No more immediately became of this, however, and Loren was relieved, worrying he or Bill had done something wrong. But in time, even as the men of the village, including the chief, began alternating between talking and singing, Loren couldn't help becoming a touch uneasy again. With his own recent experiences he had begun wondering whether the many stories he'd heard of bizarre native beliefs and rituals on this island were entirely untrue. And much as he wanted to joke with himself, right now he was at the complete mercy of those beliefs and rituals.

It was about half an hour after the chief entered, and at the end of several minutes of chanting, that Isaac startled Loren by suddenly speaking to him. Moving close he whispered, "The chief is very curious about you."

Most definitely fully awake now, Loren whispered in return, "He's curious?"

"You are not the first foreigner he has seen, but he is always curious." First glancing back at the chief, whose expression remained stern, Isaac said, "He wants to know about the place you come from. The place you told me a little about when we first talked in Wamena."

"About *Muskoka*?"

The word sounded to Loren almost alien so distant did home now seem. Also, here in surely one of the most exotic and fascinating places on earth, why would a tribal chief want to know of his plain-Jane homeland? Naturally he didn't want to raise offence with this man, but he also feared disappointing him.

"I would simply bore him," Loren at last whispered in desperation. "My home is nothing compared to his. Besides, I couldn't offer much."

Isaac shook his head. "The chief does not think so. I have told him of your lakes that can sometimes be walked on, and of tree leaves that turn many different colours. He has lived on this hilltop all his life and wants to hear more about what he sees on the horizon. And you must know this Muskoka; it is your motherland. You and this place are one and the same."

"But —"

Isaac moved and settled himself against the wall of the hut, near Loren. "Start with anything you want, and I will tell it to the chief. Start with this thing called a moose. He is very curious, and wants you to tell him everything. He says take your time — we have the whole night."

Loren again turned to the chief. He was now smiling, and by the brightness in his eyes, eagerly waiting ...

"We always thought it would be so romantic," the young woman Angela said, at the same time signalling for the waiter. "To endlessly travel the world — there's so much to experience — and to call home wherever we hung our hats for the night. Working as writers we could do it, too, what with e-mailing available almost everywhere now."

After ordering another *jugo de piña* Angela's husband, Stuart, said, "We had this great desire to break out of the stuffiness of our home town and England as a whole, to become people of the world with no specific identity other than being of this world."

"And for a while it felt like we were doing just that," Angela continued. "For almost five years we travelled non-stop. We circled the globe three times."

Loren, seated across from the couple, asked, "So what made you stop?"

Angela smiled and pointed to several other travellers who approached on the dusty road next to the restaurant. "Don't you think it's simply a hoot how some travellers dress as the locals do, thinking they'll blend in? The locals also get quite a laugh out of this, I understand. One man said to me, 'They can wear whatever they want, but we can see gringos coming from twenty miles away.'"

"I remember a day in Bolivia," Stuart quickly added, "that a farmer asked, before I had said a single word to him, and before I pulled my hood off, where in England I was from! When I asked how he so quickly knew my home country he answered in Spanish, 'Because you walk like an Englishman.' I thought — how exactly does an Englishman walk that's different from anyone else's walk, anyway? But somehow this fellow knew."

"Our point," Angela continued, "is that Stuart and I have learned something over the years. We've discovered where 'home' truly is, and where it will always be."

Stuart nodded, gazing out to the banana trees behind the patio. "The fact is — we're British. And we don't pretend to be anything but British. We know where we're from; we know of what place we're a product. We could travel forever, but Britain would still be our home. In many ways we feel like we've never left it; we've taken home with us. It's part of our luggage." Turning back to Loren, he shook his head. "No, there's no denying it. Whether or not you realize it, and whether or not you like it, the place that raised you *is* you. There's simply no denying one's roots."

Loren had entered South America in late January, flying into Caracas, Venezuela. Three and a half months later, when he met the British couple in Ecuador, he was a week from heading home.

He had seen and done much in his time on the continent. By this point in his trip he had lost considerable weight, but he still felt strong. From volcano hikes to Indian markets to river trips in the Amazon region he sensed he was collecting a near lifetime's worth of memories. Among these many experiences, however, were several that would leave especially lasting impressions.

There was, to begin, the bullfight during Ferias, or Carnival, in San Cristobal, Venezuela. Loren was invited to attend by two local men, one of whom was a schoolteacher and spoke English. "You are welcome to celebrate with us!" this man, Salvador, happily declared.

The arena proved impossibly crowded. They managed decent seats midway up the rows, however, and had a good view of the ring. From everywhere came the smell of sweat and liquor. Below them a pair of bare-chested men held a mock battle, the 'bull' repeatedly charging the shirt-wielding matador, and each time the surrounding crowd roaring "¡ole!"

The opening ceremonies had already concluded so the first fight soon began. A bull was released into the ring, and was greeted by toreros and picadors. This, Salvador explained to Loren, was the first of three *tercios*, or stages to the fight. For a quarter of an hour the toreros, sharply-dressed in bright yellow, provoked charges with their large, purplish capes, waving them at the bull and stomping their feet. At the same time the picadors, on armoured horses, also received charges and at every opportunity thrust their long pics into the bull's neck, tiring the animal and causing it to lower its head. Next the banderillos entered the ring, beginning the second tercio. They took turns planting their banderillas, or short, barbed sticks, into the bull's withers, weakening it further. Blood now streamed down its back, and Loren saw it was breathing heavily.

At last the matador, in very distinguished fashion, entered the ring. The crowd roared, and for a moment Loren could not see the ring for the many aficionados in front of him who rose to their feet. When they again settled he watched as the matador began executing a precise sequence of movements and postures that both provoked the bull and allowed a graceful escape from its charges. Again and again the matador swept his red cape, forward or backward, over the bull, stopping at times to strike a pose and acknowledge cheers from the crowd.

At last he approached the bull with a small cape, or *muleta*, in one hand and sword in the other. Standing perfectly rigid in front of the bull and aiming the sword, he lunged, and thrust the weapon into the animal's neck on his first attempt. Blood quickly began pouring from the bull's mouth. When it soon collapsed a ring assistant ran out and finished it with a knife, stabbing just behind the horns. Three elaborately-decorated horses were then used to drag the dead bull from the ring, and during this time the matador struck a final pose, accepting hearty applause.

Such repeated perhaps a dozen times that afternoon. Some matadors proved more skilled than others, but each fight ended the same. Loren consequently found it rather monotonous, and not the least sporting for the bull.

Later, while walking back through town amid the same noisy crowd, Loren questioned Salvador.

"Do you really think it's fair for the bull? Seems like it hardly stands a chance."

Salvador, frowning in a manner suggesting he had many times heard such questions, said, "Matadors do get hurt sometimes, meaning they lose, but the fight has nothing to do with fairness. You simply do not understand."

Loren dared to probe further. "But if it's not fair for both sides, how can you call it a sport. What's sporting about it?"

Salvador stopped and stared at Loren. "Bullfighting is not a sport. It is a ritual. It is ... a *dance*."

"A dance?"

Shaking his head in frustration, Salvador continued walking and offered only one last remark. "You do not know bullfighting. You must be of this place to truly understand bullfighting."

And then there had been the night in Santa Marta, Colombia. Before heading to a bar with some other travellers Loren had spoken with his hotel owner's son, a slight, fourteen-year-old named Alonzo. The boy was learning English, and wanted to practice with Loren.

The evening was clear and fresh and they took seats on an open terrace at the back of the hotel, facing the Caribbean. Alonzo's English proved already quite good, and he chatted with Loren about typical things, including school, music, and girls. Eventually, however, Loren turned conversation to the night sky, of which the terrace offered a grand view. Several days earlier he noticed Alonzo perusing an old astronomy guide from the hotel's bookshelf. He thus decided to share a particular pastime he and his father enjoyed.

One summer, when sitting on the rooftop platform at night, Loren and Stan took to learning the standard constellations. In time they became bored, however, and out of amusement began renaming them. Some of these newly-named constellations, those visible in both the northern and southern hemispheres, Loren now introduced to Alonzo.

"We call that one 'The Sagamo'," he explained, pointing out the various stars comprising what was once *Ophiuchus*, 'The Serpent Holder'. "It was a steamship back home, in the old days. You see how four stars form a box, and then another gives it a pointed end? That's the hull. The last two stars in the constellation form tie lines."

While Alonzo grinned and mused over this declaration, his father, Macario, came onto the terrace and took a seat beside him. Also able to speak English, he had heard Loren and evidently become curious. Typical of his quiet nature, he remained silent as Loren continued.

Pointing out *Aquila*, 'The Eagle', he said, "Now that one we call 'The Pike's Tooth'. Can you see it? And that one over there we've named 'The Jack Pine'." Loren pointed out what was commonly known as *Virgo*, 'The Virgin'.

He was in the midst of more when Macario suddenly spoke, cutting off his guest in mid-sentence.

"What is this silliness you are telling my son?" he asked, sternly.

Loren, surprised at this reaction, shrugged and said, "We're just having some fun. I didn't mean ..."

Macario smirked. "You think you are wise, but I have news for you. Your tree is clearly a tarantula, the fish tooth obviously a volcano, and that steamship, I will inform you, is a church. In particular, the great Santa Clara, on the Plaza Bolívar in Bogotá." Rising from his chair he added, "You have strange ideas, Señor Keswick."

Lastly had been Vilcabamba, in the very south of Ecuador, which he reached in late April. Here he spent the final week of his trip. The village was known for its relaxing atmosphere, and for the many walks it offered in the surrounding hills, including Mandango Mountain.

Loren spent most of his days partaking in such walks. He strolled the many dusty, narrow roads, and sometimes made side-trips into the neighbouring hills. He wandered for hours at a time, and almost aimlessly. Often he would end a day with the short hike to the summit of Mandango, a low mountain at the edge of the village. From here he could see for many miles in all directions, and in all those directions were rolling green hills that seemed never-ending. In the shade of a large pinnacle of rock he would seat himself to gaze at this view, and to collect his thoughts.

And by now they were troubled thoughts.

In last speaking with his mother he had professed, as usual, an eagerness for yet more travelling, but unlike past statements this time he was perhaps not telling the truth. *Perhaps* not. In this indecision lay the root of a problem only now did he realize had truly been growing from that first trip to Europe years earlier. He now saw his latest experiences in South America had only added the final touches. In short, he was not sure what he wanted to do anymore, which direction, literally or figuratively, he should head. And although part of him wondered that he simply missed home, or was merely tired, another sensed a deeper crisis, one making his mind a slurry of ideas and emotions. One afternoon during a walk he overheard a local woman, who Loren encountered numerous times, say in Spanish, "He is with San Pedro." This was an hallucinogenic cactus juice for which Vilcabamba was famous. But he was not with San Pedro, nor had he any desire to be. His thoughts were intoxicating enough; thoughts of future travels ...

He would wander forever, work as he went. He would see as much as it was possible to see. He would dive on Australia's Great Barrier reef, live with the Orang Asli of Malaysia, the Bedouin of Jordan, and the Dogon of Mali, climb Nepal's Everest and Switzerland's Matterhorn, tour the Louvre in Paris and canals of Venice, visit Machu Picchu of Peru and the Great Pyramids of Egypt, explore Namibia's Fish River Canyon, spend weeks studying rainforest butterflies in Brazil. He would climb every Ecuadorian hill he could see from Mandango Mountain. And when he died, young or old, he would die smiling. He would die not simply having existed, but having lived.

He wanted the cool lake where as a young boy he learned to swim and canoe. He wanted the white pines he and friends climbed, the smooth river stones they threw testing their aim, the birch bark they lit campfires with. He wanted to awaken to maple syrup and hemlock tea. He wanted to be remade, be renewed.

He would have friends everywhere, be welcomed in hundreds of towns and villages across the world. They would celebrate when he came. Everywhere he would be considered family.

He wanted people he knew, places he knew, food he knew, language he knew, the bed he knew, trees and rivers and birds and hills he knew.

He would write books from his experiences; he would help others in knowing the world as well as he.

He wanted to go home.

He would break away; he would be free.

He needed to go home.

On the evening he met Angela and Stuart, the British couple, at one of the village's restaurants Loren returned to his hotel late. He went straight to bed, already packed and ready to make the long bus trip to Quito in the morning. From here, several days later, he would fly to Toronto, where his parents would be waiting.

Unable to sleep in the hour that followed, liquor making him dizzy, he eventually slipped out of bed and wandered to the cabin's front window. The screen was open and the sheer white curtains rippled in the warm night air drifting in. Their edges glanced against his face as he peered out into the village's empty street. Soon, however, his gaze drifted to his new British friends, who were also still up and seated in chairs on the hotel's balcony, sheltered from a light rain that now fell. He would not join them, but leave them to the last of their travels. They too were also soon to return home.

Making his way back through the dark room to the bed he lay awake for some time before drifting into sleep. And his last thoughts were not of African highways or Asian tribal chiefs or South American star-gazings, but of home. He recalled when he was a boy, on his first camping trip in Muskoka, the night sounds, and the smell of fresh rain.

It was nearing midnight when Stan Keswick leaned forward in his chair, about to leave for bed.

"What time are you due in tomorrow?"

In the midst of yawning Loren answered, "About five."

"You plan to work those kind of hours all summer?"

"Pretty much."

"And what, dare I ask, do you plan to do with the money you put together?"

Loren offered a weak smile that on its own would have sufficed as an answer, but added, "Not for a year or so, though. And it'll be different next time."

"Seems to me it'll be the same dumb move all over again. But do as you want — it's your money, your life."

"It's a tough thing to explain, Dad. Just trust me — it'll be different next time."

There now came a clunk, the distinctive sound of the roof hatch opening. A silvery head popped up.

"Thank God — neither of you have fallen off yet. Room for an old bird?"

Stan snarled, "Don't you even think about —"

"Do as I please, old man." Mary declared firmly, casting Loren a mischievous grin. "I'm come to sit with my son." With that she gingerly stepped for the first time onto the platform, reaching for Loren's arm. Once on board she took a seat on his lap, looking rather nervous but there with him all the same.

"So? What's up?" Stan asked. "Come to rub in your own pinch of salt?"

Playfully wrapping Loren's arms around her Mary smiled. "Leave him be. The boy is back and that's all that matters. He's back where he belongs — with his dear mother."

"Which one?" Stan quipped.

And to this poke Loren could only quietly answer, "How true."

7

SUN DREAMS

The farmhouse sat on a bluff overlooking a long, open valley. At the bottom of the valley flowed a stream, and alongside it ran a narrow path which descended from the house. Upon this path one saw, looking south, rolling green pastures, the blue of a lake, and lastly, on the autumn horizon, a sliver of brilliant red and yellow maples. It was a twenty-minute walk to the lake, and the path leading to it was hard and smooth.

In the field behind the house, overgrown in long hay, sat the crumbling foundation of a barn, and next to it the tangled remains of two collapsed sheds. Although the farmhouse still stood, it too had clearly seen better days. In countless places the brickwork was cracked, the roof leaked badly, and inside, the floors rolled nearly as much as the landscape itself. And therefore no nearby resident was surprised when, the very autumn day in 1996 the farm at last changed hands, the new owners decided the house must also go.

The workers arrived in early May the following spring, a rough and tumble crew of four armed with sledgehammers, pry bars, and chain-saws. Ironically, with these tools they were to preserve as much as destroy; the antique-loving new owners decreed they salvage as much of the house's old lumber as possible for inclusion in its replacement. This made for work that was simple but tedious, and at lunch the men would laze on the long side

deck of the farmhouse, gazing silently down the valley. Occasionally soft
breezes from the distant lake drifted in, and these they welcomed.

It was on the fourth day of work one of the younger men on the crew
gutted the largest of the upstairs rooms. Determined to impress his
employer he worked quickly, and paid little attention to what he tossed
down a wooden chute leading from one of the room's windows to a fire
outside. When he happened upon a ragged book tucked behind a loose wall
board he scarcely gave it a thought.

The book struck the fire at a rapid pace and tumbled to the edge of the
pit, spilling open. This tumble offered only a temporary reprieve from the
flames; the sheer heat of the large fire would soon cause the book to ignite.
For half an hour it endured, however, the yellowed and musty pages slowly
turning, several at a time, whenever that soft lake breeze came through.
The book endured long enough that even its last pages once again saw the
light of day. And although the hand-writing filling them might have
seemed to a passing reader somewhat weak and strained, it was nonetheless
quite legible.

September 1, 1991

I woke especially early this Sunday morning. As I so wished, the
sun is shining, the grass is sparkling with dew, and the birds are
singing. How many lovely mornings such as this did we share
together in our forty-five years? You may not remember, but I do!
Mornings like this were perhaps the best thing we derived from
farming. You used to say, "Julia, this place is merely a means to an
airplane," but I'll stick with the view from the ground, thanks.

I know I haven't written to you in nearly two weeks, my dear
husband, but I've been saving and savouring, waiting for the end of
my holiday to share everything at once. My what a time I've had in
these two weeks back at the farm, and what a miracle those weeks
came about! One can, I believe, only give thanks and treasure every
moment, and this I've done.

I hope I have time to share with you all I desire to share. I don't

yet hear either of the girls stirring, but it won't be long. Little
Charlotte, surely, will be up within the hour to see her cartoons, and
I expect our daughter will also rise early on this day. Such a fuss
Brenda's made over me! It's all I can do to get her to sit down some
days. If she's not cleaning or cooking she's reading to me, especially
on those days I haven't felt up to much. What a dear she is; clearly
her father's daughter.

So many friends have called recently. I fear I'm running poor
Brenda ragged answering the phone; I am slow getting to it myself.
Many, too, have graciously taken the time to write or visit, and
some of these I want to share with you. Notably, one particularly
special 'visitor'. I feel I've almost relived my entire life in the last
few weeks so many memories have others evoked. I'm nearly at the
end of this diary, and since I intend to leave it behind (it truly
belongs with the farm), I may as well fill up the last pages. Hope you
don't mind.

The first visit I simply must tell you about is one by Nancy
Walker several weeks ago. She appeared bright and early on the
morning after I arrived at the farm, and proceeded to carry upstairs
a car load of craft supplies I had long ago given her! Before I could
stop her, insisting my hands were far too shaky nowadays to create
anything, she had pretty much set up a whole studio in the spare
bedroom. What a nut she is! A lovable nut but still a nut! She said
with so much time on my hands it would be a terrible waste of
'talent' if I wasn't creating something. The way she went on you'd
think Michelangelo had nothing on me; what friends we were
blessed with, Tom. But that's not all — what she ultimately said
made me almost fall from my chair.

It seems one evening a month earlier when the Bridge Club
girls were together the idea came up of holding an exhibit of my
works! (The drinks must have been flowing freely!) They knew the
whereabouts of most, and thought it would be interesting (and
probably amusing) to pull them together for a day and invite the
public to have a look. "It was simply an event long overdue," an
ever-smiling Nancy claimed was their thinking. And so they went
ahead. Knowing when I was visiting the farm they set up the exhibit

for my first Saturday. They were using Mavis Hall, and had planned quite an elaborate event, with music, a lunch, and speeches.

I was overwhelmed! After all these years, my first exhibit! I did consider the girls might merely be taking pity on me, but I was still flattered. Regardless, by the time Nancy left she had me committed to making an appearance at the show, and had emptied the house with what works were here. My head spun for an hour afterward.

Brenda, of course, had her concerns about me, but when my big day arrived I claimed I was feeling terrific and so she relented. Nancy came by and chauffeured her, Charlotte, and me to the hall. I felt like royalty. We arrived in plenty of time, despite a certain tiresome person pleading for a few window-gazing stops, such as when we came to the river. I couldn't believe how much my favourite little cedars had grown since I was last at the farm.

I was absolutely amazed at the number of people who attended the exhibit. When we pulled into the lot of the hall we had trouble finding a spot! I know that only means about eight cars, but still — I was again flattered. Charlotte was also evidently impressed; she ran ahead into the hall and all I heard was "My Grandma's here now!" My goodness she's something.

The afternoon went beautifully. The girls had about two dozen of the great artist's masterpieces on tables — a few hung on walls — and I saw people I hadn't seen in many years. I talked so much I started to lose my voice, and was grateful for the break when we had lunch. (And what a lovely lunch the girls put together; they had all my favourites on hand.) I also saw works I obviously hadn't seen in many years, some since doing them, and that too made for an interesting afternoon.

Do you remember Jenny Matthews? She was there, as was the piece her family commissioned for her thirtieth birthday. That must have been nearly twenty years ago. If you've forgotten, this was the Port Carling lady whose face was partly burned as a child when her mother tripped moving a pot of boiling water. She looked in good shape at the show and so did the piece. I'll refresh your memory: I took a large cast iron pot, had you drill holes in the bottom, then filled it with soil and planted marigolds. All around the outside of the pot I pasted flower show ribbons, of which Jenny had dozens. Within the forest of flowers I nestled her son's baby shoes, several of his toy cars, and a waterproofed miniature of his best-ever report card. I also tucked in a 'borrowed' pair of her husband's cuff links and a tiny photo of the couple dancing.

I was pleased to see and hear Jenny had taken good care of the piece; she kept renewing the flowers, and everything else in the arrangement also looked in fine shape. So much more did her 'pot of life' hold than hot water, and I believe Jenny has come to appreciate this. I was so happy to see her proudly smiling at the show.

Noel Ogger's piece, my largest ever, was there, although Noel himself has left us. You may remember his was the one for which I used the old 'Ogger's Bakery' sign Noel discarded when his ancient and beloved business went bankrupt. Along the edges I pasted a clipping from all the wonderful short stories he published over the years, and from the bottom of the sign I hung canes donated from the seniors' club he created. I recall this piece being considerable work; I had to have tea with Noel numerous times, quickly snatching stories from his library while he was in the kitchen. But I believe it was worth it. I heard at the show he kept the piece in his den, and continued adding stories to it up until the day he died. Good for him!

Many other works were also there, along with their owners. Verne McDonald brought his tornado-destroyed model house with protruding tree branches that sported leafy lottery winnings. Linda Grisdale brought the running shoes she wore when breaking the local mile record, the shoes (which I swiped in a frenzied run upstairs) glued to the giant collage of photos of her wheelchair-bound son. And Kathy Shaw offered the little prison I made from her family farm's mason jars, each jar holding a miniature of the high school diploma she at last received on her fiftieth birthday.

But I will not tire you with the rest. Suffice to say there was enough of my work to give me a sense of just how many pieces I had done over the years, and how many individuals were involved. Since, as you know, I never accepted payment for my works I never kept any records, and I quite honestly had lost count.

Nancy delivered us home about five, and my was I tired by that time! You would think I had jogged a hundred miles my feet were so sore. Soon after supper I slowly made my way upstairs to bed. Charlotte still came in for her story, but at Brenda's urging we kept it short on this night. I believe I was almost asleep when the two closed my bedroom door.

My first thoughts the following morning, however, were pleasant and satisfying. It had been quite a day. So often over the years I wondered whether my efforts were pointless or downright silly. No one ever said anything as such to me but then most are too polite. Seeing again, though, the people I so tried to please, so tried to offer lights of hope and celebration against their adversity, I have no regrets. All seemed to have gone on to fruitful and happy lives, and I quietly allow in my heart I played some role in that. This was all I ever wished for, not praise.

Thank you again, Tom, for tolerating my peculiar hobby all those years.

Next I want to share with you a letter from Martha Butler. I know you were not much of a fan of this lady but I would like to tell you of her letter nonetheless. She wrote to wish me well, and to tell again how much she enjoyed walking with me on and around the farm during the winter she stayed with us. I know she meant this in the sense the walks proved so helpful to me; I somehow doubt I was pleasant company at the time. She also reminded me again how understanding she was of your not wanting outside involvement in our loss, which I found comforting. How cold you were with her, Tom! Looking back with a clearer mind, I, and apparently Martha, realize you were also troubled and struggling, but how nasty you seemed at the time. I do hope now, though, you realize and accept what a wonderful gift this charming lady gave that winter, dedicating a month of her life to helping me, and truly, us.

I can not even describe to you what thoughts and feelings went through my head during the weeks following Jennifer's death. I was living in a complete blur, a life of flashes and pulses I'm unable even today to put in chronological order. As you know, as time passed I did slowly recover and was at least able to function again. But there was never complete recovery. I would like to tell you, Tom, I am today over our second daughter's death, but that would not be the truth. I know I will never be. Even now, some thirty-four years after losing her, I can still clearly picture Jennifer — the curves of her smooth, tiny face, the blue in her eyes, the shine in her long brown hair. I know you would say doing so is only to torture myself, but I'm afraid I cannot help it. I am also forever haunted by 'if onlys'. If only she had not chased that ball onto the road, if only a car had not come at that moment, if only the road was not icy that morning. Lastly, I clearly also have Charlotte as a constant reminder, so similar does she seem to Jennifer. But then, perhaps, I'm only wishing this, and I shouldn't do that. Jennifer and Charlotte are two different people. The former is gone, and all I can do is miss her very much.

Martha was so good to me for the month she stayed with us. What incredible patience and compassion she had! I wonder whether I, in a normal state, would have had the strength to deal with someone in my horrible condition at that time. Between the cooking and cleaning and attending to visitors she helped me to an extent I can never repay. And as I've mentioned, I feel particularly indebted to her for pushing me into taking long walks with her. Apparently she felt this excellent therapy, and how insightful that proved.

I don't believe I ever told of one walk she and I took — one I actually can remember clearly — since you didn't seem to much enjoy stories involving Martha. Right after she finished serving what I'm sure was a wonderful supper she drew me out the door, as usual all but putting on my coat and boots for me.

I remember the evening was cool, and we walked for some time shivering until we warmed through our exertion. Martha suggested we walk as far as the Kline farm. That was quite a distance, and I grumbled this to her. But she insisted and so on we went. This was not a new request by my partner; often she pushed me into walking long distances. I would, however, ultimately be very grateful for this particular lengthy walk.

By the time we were on the return trip from the Klines' the night seemed to have grown colder. By now Martha had run out of things to say and so we suffered this cold in silence. I do believe both of us were relieved when we at last reached our valley and the walk was almost over. It was then, however, something happened that to this day I am at a loss to explain.

Just after crossing the creek bridge a warm breeze passed through the valley from the direction of the lake. By warm I don't mean in a relative way for a cold winter night, but a *warm* breeze. Too, I swear it carried with it the scent of fresh-cut grass. Apparently I was not the only one who noticed something odd with all this, for Martha whispered to me, wide-eyed, "Well how about that!"

You may think it silly or downright unbelievable, Tom, but I believe that experience was what led me to continue with walks long after Martha returned home. I know from that evening onward I looked much more forward to such walks. Somehow I at once became more attentive to our surrounding landscape; perhaps having been blessed with such a summery surprise on that winter evening I longed for more surprises. In the years following I found them, too. Oh the lovely and fascinating walks I had, especially those along the creek to the lake! Every trip I saw something I had not seen before, from new insects to peculiar stones to plant growth and variations in the creek's course. It seemed, to sum up, the land was ever-changing, ever full of surprises and wonders. And without question my fascination helped me through mourning the loss of Jennifer. You might contend all this was merely a desperate attempt to find distraction, that I made my walk discoveries into more than they really were, but I'm not so sure. Thirty-four years later I still relish any chance to see, hear, feel, touch, or taste the land upon which we live, and much like my feelings toward Martha Butler, I feel forever indebted to it.

Brenda has just been in. Such a fuss she makes over me — have I mentioned that? Charlotte too; she brought in toast and tea, carefully placing the tray on my dresser without so much as spilling a drop. Sweet Charlotte — what a sharp little girl she is. Such a treat. Last week I helped do her hair, and she now looks lovelier than ever. How I wonder in what manner her life will unfold; she already has such grand ideas. A few days after I arrived at the farm she practically sat me down and explained her latest ambition: to become a pilot. She would build her own plane, just like she heard her grandfather wanted to, and go swooping around the whole of Muskoka, dipping now and then to visit people. It sounded so wonderful the way she described it.

Brenda has informed me the nursing home called to check on our arrival time. I readily admit (although never to Brenda) I do not look forward to returning, no offence to the home intended. I understand what my return signals the beginning of. But the reality of my illness is not to be denied, and I have no right to further burden Brenda. The work I have put her through in this two-week hiatus alone bothers me, so much do I wish to see her and Charlotte doing more lively, summery activities. Particularly Brenda; nothing would please me more than to see her patch things up with Greg, and this is clearly the best time of year for romantic thoughts. Did not two others with whom we are familiar fall in love in August?! As with our mornings at the farm, you may not remember, but I do. I suppose we can only hope for the best with our kids.

But, enough of this. On with more stories!

You'll never believe who dropped in last Sunday morning: Jack Paulie! Now there's someone I hadn't seen in quite some time. Like the rest of us he has aged, but still has a certain spring in his step. He took me completely by surprise. I was having tea in our bedroom when I heard someone on the lawn outside the window. At first I couldn't make out what the person was saying, but then I realized it was radio calls for take-offs! When I reached the window I looked down to see Jack, grinning away as usual! What a card — he's almost as nutty as Nancy Walker.

We spent the rest of the day together. The remainder of the morning we consumed looking at a handful of old photo albums Jack brought along. Many of these photos I had never seen before, and I treated each as a newfound treasure. Oh the questions I asked

Jack about them, and the stories I told after receiving my answers! I must have almost talked your poor old friend's ear off. But as you would say, "he took it like a bush pilot" and stuck with the old biddy next to him. The occasion only reinforced for me what a caring and tolerant friend you had in Jack, Tom.

Of all the photos we looked at and discussed my favourites by far were of you in, or with, Jack's little plane. One picture showed the two of you working on the engine (taken by Jack's mother), another was of you seated beside Jack in the cockpit. Lastly, many were those you took from the air. I had before seen many such photos, of course, but seeing these new ones reminded me what so thrilled and fascinated you with flying. How different the landscape looks from high above! Farmer's fields become giant quilts, forests turn to warm coats draped over the bedrock, and wide rivers become meandering, life-giving veins.

Seeing such views I again agonized over never finding the nerve to even once go up flying with Jack. I reminded him on this morning he was to take no offence at my not joining him; it was certainly not an issue of his flying skills. I'm sure you will also be pleased to hear I thanked him yet again for taking you up so many times. If Jack could only have seen his passenger, though, when he let his hair down a touch regarding planes and flying! You insisted on always being so serious and 'professional' with him. But I know different, Dear! I know the Tom who would sometimes stand on our bed in his pajamas on Saturday mornings, buzzing a small model plane through the air while I lay watching below. And the one who sometimes used me as a landing strip! But I mustn't go into that. Suffice to say flying, even if it wasn't you at the controls, was one truly great gift you received in life, my dear husband, and I believe you should always remember that.

We had lunch on the side deck, one which Brenda so kindly made for us. As we ate I looked out over this valley we were so blessed with. When Jack suggested we were also cursed with it, however, I had difficulty arguing. How tough a time we truly had with farming.

One might now chuckle over some of the things we did to

make ends meet — the many and sometimes odd jobs in town we took — but at the time I don't recall any such chuckles. When I think of the sort of hours you especially put in to keep the farm and us alive I almost shudder. All I can say is I'm happy we managed to shield our kids from these hardships, or at least for the most part. When I occasionally speak with Brenda about her 'old days' on the farm she sometimes comes out with comments making me wonder just how shielded she was. Often, it seems, she was kidded at school about her small and modest wardrobe. When she speaks of this she invariably laughs, but once again, I somehow doubt she laughed at the time. She also sometimes makes a joke out of how spare some of our family occasions were, and these stories I find particularly painful. We struggled badly in making birthdays, for instance, special days for the girls. Although some will argue "family is all that's really important," I believe the reality is, young girls want *things*. They want toys and dresses and shoes. And it pains me deeply we could offer them so little.

Jack, it seems, knew of our troubles quite well.

He told me a story about a day he helped you make some repairs to the barn. Several boards had blown off high up on the south end, and you needed a hand holding the new ones in place so you could nail them. Jack said every time you drove a nail, however, the modest lumber only split, and eventually you had to tear both pieces off, leaving a large hole again. He also told me, I hope you don't mind, that you spent almost the next twenty minutes with your head in your hands. He told me he had never before seen you that upset, and this was when he first realized how tough a time we, and especially you, were having. The boards may have been but a small problem on their own, but he knew they were merely one on a long list. A list that would likely have broken most men. But as Jack said during our day, when you at last rose and continued work he was at once in awe of you. He said he would trade his pilot's license any day of the year for backbone like yours. I was quite touched.

Late that fine afternoon we took a drive to Nathan's. It seemed only fitting after spending the entire day talking about you. When we arrived I was a little surprised that Jack knew so well where you were, but shouldn't have been. He was as close a friend to you as I think anyone, Tom.

Your marker I've kept tidy, you'll be happy to know, and I would like to refresh your memory of what is engraved on its face:

Thomas Stanley Neal
1915-1984

Here lies the finest husband one could ever hope for
A man of determination
A man of love and generosity
May he at last lie in peace

We stood silently at your grave what I'm sure were only several minutes. In those few minutes, however, a flood of memories passed through me: of the two of us on our first date, of our wedding day, of the days Brenda and Jennifer were born, of you holding Charlotte when she was only a year old, and lastly, of you warmly holding my hand the day you died. Too, as we soon returned to the car Jack pointed out a small airplane moving gracefully across the sky. At that moment I could also see you up there, up flying that great bird yourself, and joyously waving down at me.

I miss you so much, Tom.

Brenda has just been in again, this time to help me pack my things so she can start loading the car. I hope I don't sound cynical, but I wondered at some of the items we packed; I might prefer having many of my belongings simply left at the farm. I know I've already mentioned this, but I will tell you again I intend to leave this diary behind. To me it belongs here, at home, and when the day comes the house leaves this world then so too should this diary. When I finish writing to you today I will therefore store the book in its usual spot. And since you accidentally saw me doing so one day decades ago, I know darn well you're familiar with that spot! You were so kind not to admit this, though, and also so considerate not to read what I wrote before you passed. I always tucked a tiny piece of thread inside the front cover, and never found it missing. You're such a dear.

I do believe I have just enough time to share with you what I've been secretly leading up to all this time — the events of last Wednesday afternoon!

They effectively began while I sat in the front porch after lunch. Little Charlotte quietly stepped in and asked a question taking me quite by surprise. She inquired if I had time for *her* to visit me now! Oh how I felt guilty! With getting so many letters and phone calls, and with so many people dropping by, it seems I was neglecting the visitor most precious to me of all. Instantly I resolved to make it up to her.

Brenda went shopping that afternoon, and with her not present to stop me I summoned all my strength and took a stroll with our dear granddaughter into the valley. It was slow going for me, of course, but the little bundle in front — my goodness! I think she did four miles worth of circles and tumbles by the time we reached the creek. Watching her brought tears to my eyes I was so thrilled.

An hour passed quickly. We watched and spoke with minnows in the creek, had a very one-sided game of tag, then sat together in the field. I gingerly settled myself down while Charlotte simply fell back into the long grass, giggling away. For the first time since we left the house she then actually stayed relatively still for a while.

The day was delightful. The sun was shining, but now in late summer it was not as hot as earlier. That occasional but ever-present breeze from the lake, too, was cool and refreshing. What really made the afternoon, however, were the wildflowers! On both sides of the valley, including where we sat near the creek, goldenrods and purple asters had taken over, and how! I know you will not be impressed to hear such 'weeds' have blanketed your hard-worked fields for many autumns now. Please forgive me, then, when I say they were truly a sight to behold.

Now it was after describing to Charlotte how much plainer the fields once looked, before she was born, that she gave me a second surprise on this day. Even more of one, for what she said would keep me thinking for days. Indeed I still am.

Running her tiny fingers over one of the purple asters, Charlotte said, "If the fields were plain, then maybe these flowers are something the sun dreamed up to make you happy, Grandma."

I smiled at her. "Something the sun dreamed up?"

"Sure. Everybody else dreams up stuff. You make stuff up for people, like your sculpture things, so maybe the sun decided to decorate this field with flowers for you."

Have you ever heard such a notion?!

I must admit I initially thought nothing of it, myself; like all kids her age Charlotte often comes up with peculiar ideas. But during the evening of that day, and indeed since that afternoon, I have been captivated by this particular notion, musing over it for hours. I would like to share such thoughts with you.

Silly as it may at first sound, but I began wondering, Tom, if our eight-year-old granddaughter's idea might hold a message for me, and for you; a key to making sense of all we've been through in our lives. If, after all, a field of wildflowers is a creative, well-intentioned endeavour of the sun, or of some other all-encompassing power, then so perhaps might our entire landscape and all that goes on within it. And just like all mortal artists including myself, this artist is forever experimenting, forever learning, forever caught between satisfaction and dissatisfaction, pleasing and displeasing. I also don't know whether you feel the same, but considering the world and our lives in this light — as a grand and endless experiment by a well-meaning but imperfect creator — I find comforting. To me it invites tolerance and forgiveness for the misfortunes we've suffered, and wonder and celebration over that which we've been blessed. Like our children, like our farm, like, truly, our fields of goldenrods and purple asters.

I can only imagine what new ideas Charlotte's sun may dream up for this valley. Perhaps, one day in the distant future, it may decide on it not being a valley at all; great mountains may again rise here, or perhaps the land is to be covered by ocean, or desert, or rainforest. The sky, according to Charlotte, is the limit. The sun's palette is apparently infinite. And what, too, might it dream up for those who live within this landscape? What fortunes and misfortunes, for instance, will unfold for Brenda, or for dear Charlotte? I may never know, but I find a certain comfort in the notion their fate, marked by ups and downs as it may be, is at least a well-intentioned fate. And I hope you find comfort in this too, Tom. I love you so much.

But oh my goodness! How quickly the morning has passed! I've just checked the window again and I see Brenda has finished loading the car. Soon she'll be up for me, so I will close and tuck this diary away once and for all. As you know, Brenda would never press, Tom, but I shouldn't keep her waiting. She's been so wonderful. Too, I doubt the view from my window could ever be more lovely than it is at this moment: the lake, the valley, and from the car, dear Charlotte smiling up at me.

Epilogue

The evening was a fine one, was the consensus. Overcast and windy through most of the day, the sky had cleared to a deep blue and the air was now still. At Bracebridge Bay several thousand year-round residents, cottagers, and tourists have gathered under an early moon, filling the grassy parks on both sides, awaiting the Kinsmen's summer fireworks. It is July 1; Canada Day.

There are faces here familiar to you. A retired Jim and Doris Stanford are seated in souvenir lodge chairs in the south park, Jim nodding at regular intervals with passing former guests, Doris silently branding. The entire Stanton Corner crew are also here, arriving having spent the afternoon welcoming a new singer. Loren Keswick has recently returned to "both his mothers" from yet another trip abroad, and has just made a purchase from 'Doug & Ronnie's SuperDogs', curiously tucked into the bush behind the tennis courts. In the northern park is an eighteen-year-old Charlotte Warren, her eyes aglow with a grandmother's wonder, while Jack Bennett treats a visiting grandson to 'The Bracebridge Bay Sandbar: A Steamship Captain's Nightmare'. Lastly, Fred Sutton and his daughter Christina are here. Fred, you may be happy to know, is enjoying yet another splendid cottaging summer, forgetful still of those long past, but cherishing the present.

Among the many others gathered on this evening are countless more stories of Muskoka that could be told. Faces offer clues to facets of this land past and present, but also of the future. And similarly across the country, and across the world, are such faces, each harbouring its own story of a particular home, and, perhaps unknowingly, a story of that greater home all share. Each, as Lorna Steinberg would say, lending a unique sparkle to the same precious stone.

Also By Robert Rea

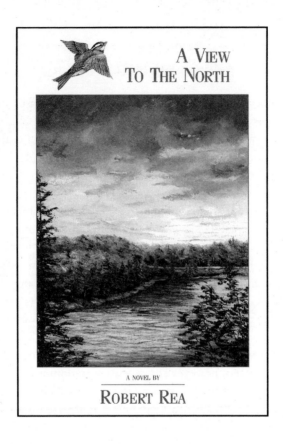

A VIEW
TO THE NORTH

A NOVEL BY

ROBERT REA

Muskoka's Best-selling Novel for 2000!

Now in Second Print

Written with humour, compassion, and insight, *A View To The North* explores what may proved the most complex and debated topic of this new century — the human relationship with wild nature.

When Bruce and Valerie Farrow move their city-raised family from Toronto to the wilds of Muskoka, their ten-year-old son worries this dramatic lifestyle change will prove turbulent — and his worries are soon justified. Reflecting as an adult, Lewis Farrow recounts the triumphs and tragedies of his earliest years living on a tiny Muskoka lake, and how the surrounding woods and colourful lake residents profoundly influence his later life. With an informal, down-to-earth narrative that ranges from humorous to heart-wrenching, *A View To The North* explores the complexities of the human relationship with 'Mother Nature'.

"Rea writes from experience when he places his novel in a Muskoka setting and catches all the nuances of its many-sided personality ... an excellent read. Get a copy and curl up."
Judith Ruan, *Muskoka Magazine*

"Rea's characters [are] realistic and enduring ..."
Eleanor Kidd, *The Huntsville Forester*

"... a stimulating Muskoka read, but its readership needn't be restricted to this neck of the woods."
Cathy Cahill-Kuntz, *The Muskokan*

ADDITIONAL COPIES

To obtain copies of any MapleLand Press book, please check your local bookstore, or order directly from:

MapleLand Press
P.O. Box 1285
Bracebridge, Ontario
Canada
P1L 1V4

SUN DREAMS
Robert Rea
Can. $14.95, U.S. $11.95

A VIEW TO THE NORTH
Robert Rea
Can. $18.95, U.S. $14.95

For single-book orders, please add
Can. $4.00 (U.S. $ 3.00) shipping and handling.

For multiple-book orders, please add
Can. $4.00 (U.S. $ 3.00) shipping and handling
for first book plus Can. $0.75 (U.S. $0.50) per extra book.

Payable by cheque or money order.
In Canada and the U.S., please allow up to four weeks for delivery. Elsewhere up to six weeks.